# Continuity of Nursing Care

Edited by
**Sue K Armitage**
Formerly All Wales Research Liaison Nurse
Cardiff

With Eight Contributors

Foreword by
**C A Butterworth**
Queen's Nursing Institute Professor of Community Nursing
University of Manchester

**Scutari Press**
London

Scutari Press is a division of Scutari Projects Ltd,
the publishing company of the Royal College of Nursing

First published 1991

**British Library Cataloguing in Publication Data**

Continuity of nursing care.
　1. Medicine. Nursing
　I. Armitage, Sue K.
　610.73


ISBN 1-871364-48-5

Typeset by Blackpool Typesetting Services Limited
Printed and bound by Page Bros (Norwich) Ltd.

# Continuity of Nursing Care

# Contributors

SUE K ARMITAGE PhD BA(Hons) RGN
Formerly All Wales Research Liaison Nurse, South Glamorgan Health Authority

DENISE E BARNETT BA(Hons) SRN SCM RCNT Dip N(Lond)
Formerly District Adviser (Nursing and Quality Assurance), West Essex Health Authority

ROGER DEEKS BA RGN RNT CertEd
Sub-Unit Manager, Gloucester Health Authority Community Unit

BRIDIE LUIS FUENTES RGN RM RHV
Health Visitor, Gwent Health Authority

SARAH JOWETT MSc BNurs RGN RHV DN
Health Visitor, Trafford Health Authority

MARGARET MACDONALD MN MA RGN SCM
Coordinator of the Scottish Nursing Standards Project

CLARE NEWMAN RGN NDN
Community Nursing Sister, Mid Glamorgan Health Authority

JAN M O'LEARY SRN ONC NDN CertPWT
Manager, Hospital/Community Liaison and Support Services, West Suffolk Health Authority

FELICITY A WATSON SRN NDN
Nursing Officer for District Nursing, Nurse Adviser (Community), West Cumbria Health District

# Contents

# Acknowledgements

My thanks are due to the contributing authors for their readiness to submit manuscripts and to Lesley Player for her help in compiling the volume.

# Foreword

Health care provision has to span the complexities of a many layered system. To be effective this provision must have some system of continuity across the very real service divisions which exist between public health care services, primary health care, specialist hospital provision and residential services.

This book is a most welcome addition to the literature on this important debate. Edited by a nurse with considerable research expertise in the subject area, the book refocuses our attention on the thorny problem of maintaining dialogue between these services and, more importantly, with consumers of the services.

It offers fresh information, which lends new strength to the case for effective liaison between nursing services, much of which has been generated from a substantial research project carried out by the editor in a national study. The various responsibilities of the actors involved in the process of liaison are reviewed by authors with considerable experience in liaison, management practice and research. It is easy to see that this book will become an important source of reference for all nurses in community and hospital settings who struggle to provide some sense of continuity between the different services involved. As nurse education across the world begins to prepare nurses for 'Health for All by the Year 2000', new types of nurses must emerge, who are capable of bridging the gaps so clearly identified in this book.

We owe to ourselves and to those for whom we care, to improve upon continuity of care. This book will help us to help ourselves and I recommend it to all those involved which must, inevitably, include us all.

Tony Butterworth 1991

# Preface

Continuity of nursing care implies the coordinated and uninterrupted provision of care that is suited to patients' needs, but, in reality, general nursing care is usually split and provided in hospital and at home by two different groups of nurses. The interface between hospital and community has been an area of concern for many years and in recent times the decrease in patients' length of stay in hospital, coupled with the increase in the numbers of elderly patients, has inevitably increased the burden of caring in the community.

We live in a time of continuous change both in the organisation and delivery of the health service and in the education of nurses, midwives and health visitors. The provision of care across boundaries has never been easy, and realistic packages of care will need to be negotiated to take into account the health and social needs of patients in different settings. Discharge planning will become an increasingly important element of an effective service. As the education of nurses will, in future, prepare them for practice in both hospital and the community, it is important to examine the underlying key issues that affect the continuity of day-to-day nursing care in order to be able to understand where change is required.

Much can be learnt from nurses who have experience of maintaining care between hospital and home, and in this volume district nurses, health visitors and hospital nurses, together with their managers, discuss the factors that affect and influence the continuity of nursing care. Tried and tested solutions to problems in various situations are presented.

This book is intended for all who need to consider the provision of continuing hospital and community care of patients, for those doing the job now in a changing situation, for those who will educate students to work in both places, the students themselves, and for the managers of the services. It is time again to focus on patient care between the two areas of hospital and home.

Sue Armitage 1991

# 1
# Introduction

Sue Armitage

---

Nursing care is provided in both hospital and home, but not by the same group of nurses. For two decades we have been aware that patients who return to their own homes from hospital are not always cared for in a continuous manner (Hockey, 1968; Skeet, 1970). What happens between hospital and home is of crucial concern to the patient. The experience of being cared for can be perceived as broken or as continuous between the two areas. Many hospital patients may feel ready to return home, both physically and emotionally, and yet find that they are weaker and less able to cope at home than they had anticipated. Others, especially the elderly who live alone, may wish to stay a little longer within the sheltered environment of a hospital where meals, warmth, and company are provided without their effort. But beds are in short supply and the elderly who live alone must often return to their homes before they feel ready. The period of readjustment is crucial to any person's well-being. It is a nursing function to ensure that care is continued during the period when most patients feel particularly vulnerable after a stay in hospital and until home life is re-established; yet this crucial area of care falls between hospital nurses and community nurses.

Not every patient who leaves hospital needs professional community care and support services. Many patients – the elderly among them – will be cared for by family or friends (Garrett, 1985). Fundamental questions need to be addressed to determine why it remains such a problem to ensure that care is unbroken. The National Health Service is a large, bureaucratic organisation with many different sections operating within it, and little in the way of an overview. Overall account is rarely taken of differences in day-to-day working so that these different sections can be effectively co-ordinated. For the hard-pressed worker immediacy is the keynote, and effecting change outside the boundaries of everyday working contacts an impossibility.

The middle manager can exercise a certain level of power to effect change but if he/she is unaware of problems that are lived with on a daily basis rather than articulated, change will not take place. An overview, in the form of an organisational cross-section of different levels of working, is required in order to examine the functioning of a number of cells that interact only peripherally.

The perspective given by professionals of their role in continuity of care is almost invariably partial. The picture gained of liaison in general from hospital nurses in Melia and Macmillan's study is one of 'organisational formality rather than a means of facilitating continuity of care' (1983: p.155).

It is often said that district nurses have the advantage of hospital nursing experience before working in the community. In rare instances they then return to work in hospital or hold integrated posts (Jowett and Armitage, 1988). The starting point, though, is with the normative ideology of hospital care although nursing education in the future will shift this focus (UKCC, 1987).

## HISTORICAL BACKGROUND

We need to ask why many of the problems that existed in Hockey's account of district nursing care on discharge (Hockey, 1968), still pertain even after the implementation of a number of National Health Service reorganisations introduced to coordinate different parts of the service. When Hockey conducted her study hospital and community health services were administered separately, and it is perhaps more understandable to find that hospital consultants were reluctant to refer patients to community care and were uncertain about what this involved, simply because they were unaware of what services existed and the form in which they were available. But delays and inadequacies identified by Hockey in both medical and nursing reports sent from hospital to community staff still exist (Mageean, 1986). Nursing referral forms were found to be inadequate, and years later work still continues in an effort to develop appropriate documentation (Skeet, 1980; Garrett, 1985; Gilchrist, 1987).

Just two years after Hockey published her findings, Skeet (1970) investigated what patients saw their home-care needs to be. The number of community services called upon within the first two weeks of discharge were double the number arranged by hospital staff. This implies that patients were not adequately or realistically assessed for home support while still in hospital, and that responsibility for arranging aftercare was not seen as an important function of the role of staff in hospital.

Roberts' study (1975) was similarly concerned with the problems of discharge and set out to measure the effectiveness of care experienced by people recently discharged from hospital. A tentative conclusion drawn from the results was that age had little to do with the prediction of aftercare needs and yet this is one of the criteria frequently given for referring patients to aftercare services (Armitage, 1979).

One of the purposes of the 1974 NHS reorganisation was the improvement of hospital/community liaison by combining them under one administrative umbrella – the Area Health Authorities (DHSS, 1972). Since that time, there has been little evidence to suggest that this was effective. A number of studies undertaken by Age Concern in the mid- and late 1970s focused on the needs and care of elderly patients after discharge from hospital. In the main, they found the same problems occurring in the post-discharge period when the patient returns home, often to an ill-prepared situation, owing to a lack of awareness about the importance of identifying needs early enough for arrangements to be made (Amos, 1973; Age Concern, 1975; Slack and Gibbins, 1979; Thurstans, 1980; Skeet, 1982).

Coinciding with the 1982 NHS reorganisation (Chaplin, 1982), there was a marked increase in the number of jobs advertised for liaison nurses to work between hospital and community. There was no direct recommendation leading to this move, but over ten years' research had certainly pointed towards a need. Despite a wealth of evidence identifying specific problems, these had not been remedied.

The problems of ensuring continuing care are well documented for their complexity (Armitage, 1979, 1981; Cass, 1978; Amos, 1973; Skeet, 1980, 1982; Hockey, 1968; Simpson and Levitt, 1981). Roberts (1975) recognised that the studies concentrating on the discharge point from hospital tackled only one facet, and that the many prior events affect what happens when a patient leaves hospital.

## REFERRAL FOR DISCHARGE

A study of the assessment and planning stages for discharge showed a number of discrepancies between what professionals said should happen and what actually did happen (Armitage, 1979).

The main criteria used to refer patients to hospital, social and voluntary services were elicited from nurses, doctors, social workers, physiotherapists and occupational therapists. The stated criteria for referral in many instances did not match the actual criteria used in relation to identified particular patients, even when a liaison nurse was involved. Jowett and Armitage (chapter 6 this volume) describe in detail the complexity and disparity in the role of liaison nurses and clearly illustrate the difficulties of those who do not have day-to-day contact with patients for whom arrangements are being made.

Patient care is a complicated business always subject to influences affecting its delivery. Discharge is not a single event when a patient leaves hospital but is a stage in patient care situated on a continuum which has a period of preparation and from which consequences ensue (Armitage, 1981). Attempts have been made to move away from allusion to the single event of leaving hospital, as if all it entails is walking out of the ward, by referring to 'transfer' of patients between hospital and home. Unfortunately, this is often misunderstood and is still largely used when patients are transferred between and within hospital services.

For hospital staff – both nursing and medical – the norms are still those of the patient in hospital and not of the patient in the context of the home environment (Dartington, 1974). This reflects the way in which both nurses and doctors have been taught to perceive patients. In the future this will change (UKCC, 1987) and already, in many instances, changes in nurse education have been made. A community perspective will be included, but with many current hospital staff having little community experience, the problem remains. Until a hospital stay is seen only as an interlude for a person whose real life exists outside the hospital, the patient will dominate the person. It is unrealistic to expect nurses, who have had little experience of community nursing themselves, to be able to impart to students on their ward a perspective of continuing patient care they do not possess. Similarly, few nurse teachers with district nursing qualifications specialise in teaching on a Registered General Nurse (RGN) programme. The community perspective, like research, may often be an add-on element in the curriculum rather than integrated within it.

The notion of patient assessment, whether as part of a medical, nursing or social diagnosis, is complex, for it takes into account not only the physical condition of the patient but the psychosocial factors as well. Knowledge of the patient's home and social circumstances is fundamental to understanding the effect on a patient of both admission to hospital and return home. Unless prime responsibility is taken for a total assessment by one individual who is experienced not only in eliciting the right sort of information but who can also communicate it verbally and in written form, then a true nursing assessment will not be forthcoming. The alternative will be a partial attempt to understand the effects of ill health on the total patient.

Patient assessment may – but does not necesssarily – imply subsequent action. Armitage (1979) analysed the referrals made before medical patients were discharged. They fell into the four categories of completed, missed, abortive and intended referrals. In a sample of 80 medical in-patients (40 male and 40 female) 11 men (27.5 per cent) and 16 women (40 per cent) were referred for continuing care

**Table 1.1  Categories of referral**

| To | Missed | Intended | Abortive | Completed | Total |
|---|---|---|---|---|---|
| Social worker | 6 | 2 | 2 | 12 | 22 |
| Health visitor | 5 | – | – | 12 | 17 |
| District nurse | – | – | – | 6 | 6 |
| Physiotherapist | – | 2 | 1 | 8 | 11 |
| Occupational therapist | – | – | 1 | 1 | 2 |
| Total | 11 | 4 | 4 | 39 | 58 |

services. Eleven patients were referred to more than one agency.

The category of *completed referrals* was made and carried through, although the final outcome was not necessarily explored if a visit had not been made, for example, by the health visitor, at the time the patient was interviewed at home 7–10 days after discharge. What was known was that the referral had been received. The moot point in considering the category of 'completed referrals' is whether or not it matters that a visit had not been made within ten days of the patient leaving hospital. The fundamental question of the role of health visiting in post-discharge and continuing care is raised. General surveillance versus particular assessment visits require different timing. If patients are expecting a visit it is important that they should have a general idea of its purpose and when to expect it. Uncertainty is increased by hospital nurses' lack of understanding of the role of the health visitor in relation to the elderly (Melia and Macmillan, 1983; Armitage, 1989).

In the second category of *missed referrals*, patients fitted the referral criteria stated by professionals but these did not, in practice, take place. For example: 'We always refer diabetic patients to the health visitor', or 'We always refer patients over 75 who live alone to the district nurse', but in practice no referral had been made.

Thirdly, the category of *abortive referrals* described referrals which were made but which for some reason were not carried through. For example, a nurse might have initiated a referral but a physician felt it to be either inappropriate or premature and so nothing further was done. The referral criteria were therefore obviously not shared by nurse and doctor and the latter determined what was considered appropriate. The person who received the referral – for example, the social worker – was then involved in wasted time and effort, the amount depending on how far the referral had gone before it was stopped.

The final and fourth category of *intended referrals* described those instances where the ward sister, or perhaps the social worker, said a referral would be made but where in practice nothing was done, often because it was decided that the patient would be discharged. The numbers are small but reflect a worrying trend when it is realised that for 80 patients studied and 58 referrals made, 33 per cent of them (19) did not come to fruition. Nineteen per cent (11) were missed.

Criteria given by professionals are insufficient to predict whether or not a referral is made and even less, whether it is completed. The referral process consists of an often lengthy and complex series of events and it is not easy to generalise about it. There are no hard-and-fast criteria relating to assessment of perceived needs of patients. A lack of communication between staff can result in a haphazard pattern of referral and alter the outcome for patients.

## PATIENT ASSESSMENT

Various terms such as nursing assessment, nursing diagnosis (Draper, 1986) or social diagnosis (Richmond, 1917) attempt to label an often lengthy process. Patients' felt need may not be expressed or match the professionals' sense of normative need (Bradshaw, 1972). Patients may be so relieved to be discharged home that they and their relatives suppress any misgivings they have about their ability to manage at home. A hospital nurse or doctor with experience confined to that situation will see that the patient is able to manage in hospital. It is a different matter for an elderly, infirm patient at home with an equally elderly spouse and without hospital laundry facilities, the provision of meals and so on.

An individualised assessment takes account not only of physical needs but also of patients' social circumstances. If the patient is assessed purely in physical terms then only those referrals will be made that are necessary to maintain the physical status quo. Patients admitted with an acute exacerbation of an existing condition are more likely to be discharged to the same home situation, even if that is what contributed to their illness. Unless all patients are assessed as a matter of course, using social as well as physical criteria, only patients whose physical condition would be changed on discharge are guaranteed a more comprehensive assessment.

There are times when both relatives' and nurses' protestations about patients' unreadiness to return home are overruled, usually by medical staff who wish to ensure bed availability and a faster patient throughput. It has been shown (Armitage, 1981) that a covert negotiation of patients' needs presented by nurses and junior doctors to senior medical staff most effectively achieves what patients want in the long run, especially when they say that they do not feel well enough to return home.

## NURSING PROCESS

The introduction of nursing process appeared to offer the solution to many of the disjointed problems of patients' assessment. Introduced to the United Kingdom from the United States in the late 1960s and early 1970s, it advocated a systematic and holistic approach to individualised patient care and the opportunity to make explicit, systemise and document the way in which many 'good' nurses felt they had been caring for patients for years. Broadly consisting of the four stages of assessment, planning, intervention and evaluation, nursing process demanded the explicit separation of each of these stages in a new and hitherto undocumented form. The existing nursing reports were to be superseded by nursing process documentation allowing the identification of nursing problems following a systematic assessment.

Much has been written about the failure of the approach in its early stages (Nicklin, 1984; Wright, 1985a). It was largely introduced not as a concept to aid the way in which nursing care could be thought about, organised and delivered, but as a new set of forms which had to be completed in a different way from the old while nursing care was given in the same task-centred way.

The ideology of holistic, individualised care demands not only the patient's own participation in care but the inclusion of the family in the patient's care too, and in that way recognition of the factors affecting the social environment and home life. The emphasis therefore moves away from the patient's medical diagnosis and physical symptoms to the care of the total person. With the advent of nursing process, nursing had come of age with the acceptance and overt acknowledgement of its unique, continuous function.

In reality, much remained the same, with increasing frustration over the amount of additional paperwork and little change in practice. The ideological foundation, with a consideration of its underlying concepts was not explored, mainly because those who introduced nursing process did not themselves understand its requirements to reorganise nursing care in a problem-oriented way this rested not on nursing care required for a medical diagnosis but elicited an assessment of what the illness or condition meant to the patient and how nursing skills could be used to care and help understanding of a condition. The detailed knowledge required to care for patients in this way requires documentation to ensure continuity of care.

Before the advent of nursing process, nurses had never been encouraged to spend time writing a nursing record, especially one which required careful thought and a systematic approach. Nursing process demands a staging of care, culminating in the evaluation of whether or not the planned and delivered care is considered to be effective. This approach is certainly something that nurses find difficult and with which they struggle.

Nurses in Britain are not alone, it seems, in their difficulties in comprehending the semantic vagaries of nursing innovations. Webb (1984) described to overseas colleagues the dilemma in which nurses who advocate nursing theories and the use of nursing process, claiming them as the routes of professional status and high quality care, were being directly opposed by the 'doers' of nursing. The latter's claims were concerned with the incomprehensibility of the language used, especially in certain of the nursing models (Wright, 1985b, 1986) and their total lack of a contribution to the day-to-day delivery of nursing care (Luker, 1988). Webb (1984) found similar difficulties had been experienced by North American nurses who are now questioning the status of nursing theories which are largely seen to be unsubstantiated by research and more appropriately viewed as a lower-order 'conceptual framework', if used at all. British nurses are travelling along a similar road to their US colleagues. Webb describes their moves to use nursing diagnosis not as another theory but as a way of ensuring a systematic approach to care which focuses on nursing as a distinct discipline from medicine.

In short, a definitive approach to nursing care has not yet been reached and there is still a need constantly to question, criticise and try new approaches.

## COMMUNITY REPORTS

A plethora of recent reports have focused specifically on community care with varying mention of continuing services between hospital and home, although each has implications for it. Community nursing has come into the limelight with a number of reviews in recent years.

In England, the first community nursing review was published following a six-month undertaking by a working party (DHSS, 1986a, the Cumberlege Report). It introduced the concept of 'neighbourhood nursing' for planning, organising and providing primary care. In place of existing district nurse and health visitor attachment to general practices and health centres, each neighbourhood nursing service, headed by a nurse manager, would include a care team, comprising district nurses, health visitors and school nurses. They would work closely with primary health care teams, reinforcing them but not substituting for them. Other community nurses, such as midwives, psychiatric nurses and mental handicap nurses, would coordinate their work with the neighbourhood nursing services through their own managers.

Despite some opposition initially from general practitioners, and often without waiting for specific government approval of the contents of the report, moves were made towards restructuring the services.

A function of the community nursing services was seen to be the avoidance of hospital admission, as well as facilitation of early discharge, by working with informal carers. In order to monitor and improve community nursing services, a checklist was suggested for health authorities to keep under regular review. In relation to coordination of services, 'There should be clearly understood arrangements between hospital and community nursing staff concerning the admission to hospital and discharge of patients to ensure adequate support is available on their return' (DHSS, 1986a, p.12).

Soon after the English community nursing review was published, a discussion document on primary health care (DHSS, 1987) was released which largely reinforced the general conclusions reached in the Cumberlege Report.

In the government white paper 'Promoting Better Health' (DHSS, 1987) comments on the Cumberlege Report recommendations were made and it was reported that the House of Commons Social Services Committee's report on primary health care gave a 'cautious welcome to the proposals for establishing community nursing in smaller units based on defined populations' (DHSS, 1987, p.70). By 1988, many districts in England had proceeded with the introduction of neighbourhood nursing (*Nursing Standard*, 1988).

A further government-commissioned community report (Griffiths, 1988) placed emphasis on local authority provision of services. Little mention was made of community nursing services other than that recommendations made may affect but not diminish their contribution and that 'the special skills of community nurses should be used to best effect' (p.15). Within a framework of flexibility concerning who does what, 'the professional skills of community nurses and health visitors need to be effectively harnessed' (p.25).

The subject of continuing care was dealt with mainly in relation to patients discharged from mental hospitals who should have a 'package of care devised' and be the responsibility of a 'named care worker' (p.v).

Acute hospital services and community care were seen to be complementary and with interaction between them: 'In some cases there may be a need to improve planning and communication between different bodies, so that the appropriate range of services is readily available to patients when they are discharged from hospital' (p.8).

The Welsh community nursing review (Edwards, 1987) was published after a wide-ranging two-year consultation by the review team with health professionals from all disciplines, as well as actual and potential consumers and their carers. The scale and range of community nursing was recognised in the context of the complex networks within which it operates.

With reference specifically to the links between hospital and community, the evidence to the review team showed up the 'initial absence of liaison between hospital and community' (p.50). Where it did exist, usually in relation to care of the elderly, the amount of time spent on clerical work was recognised. The difficulties created by the absence of equipment to ease and aid communication (e.g. answering machines at nursing bases and two-way radios or radio pagers) were acknowledged. The recommendation was made that 'liaison staff employed in the community health services and with considerable community experience be attached to acute hospitals' (p.50). Subsequently, in a Departmental circular (WHC(89)23) giving guidance to the future development for the recommendations of the Welsh Community Nursing Review, this recommendation was reiterated.

The community nursing review for Northern Ireland (DHSS, 1986b) stated: 'It is not considered necessary for the post of Liaison Nurse to be continued' (pp.167, 344) and that local review of liaison arrangements by directors of nursing services should be undertaken to ensure that discharge procedures ensured continuity of nursing care. Direct liaison between hospital and community nurses was encouraged as well as the exchange and provision of bilateral information on both admission to hospital of patients known to community nurses and at discharge with a discharge summary. Induction programmes and in-service training for all hospital and community staff should include the subject of hospital/community liaison arrangements.

A much welcomed health circular (HC(89)5) concentrates entirely on the discharge of patients from hospital. It emphasises the importance of a multidisciplinary approach to early discharge planning beginning soon after admission to hospital and before admission for those patients whose admissions are planned and for whom it is known support will be needed after returning home. Patients themselves, together with their family and other carers, are appropriately placed at the centre of the planning process.

A checklist is recommended to ensure the completion of arrangements and the recommendation made that it should be retained in the patient's notes as a 'permanent record of action taken before discharge'. The responsibility of checking adequate discharge preparation should be given to one specific member of staff caring for that patient, the professional discipline being unspecified. Emphasis is on the importance of multidisciplinary collaboration. Health authorities are recommended to review existing discharge procedures in wards and departments in consultation with all those involved.

A booklet issued at the same time gives guidelineṡ intended for those drawing up discharge procedures to meet the requirements of the health circular (DoH, 1989). Attention is drawn to those likely to need specific arrangements such as the elderly living alone, the terminally ill, the chronically disabled and mothers of babies in special or intensive care. The importance of involving community nursing services in pre-discharge planning, either directly or through a community liaison sister, is recognised, and that the community nursing staff visiting a patient in hospital and having discussions with the ward sister may avoid later problems.

A local authority circular issued in conjunction with the health circular and an accompanying guidance booklet on discharge seek a similar review of existing procedures and arrangements (LAC(89)7). The importance of joint planning with health services is emphasised in order to maintain patients who need continuing care in their home.

## DISCHARGE PLANNING

In the US attention is being paid to discharge planning as a discrete activity of patient care (McKeehan, 1981; McClelland et al., 1985). It is identified as the *process* by which the *goal* of continuity of care is attained (Buckwalter, 1985). Time and again, authors point to the need for multi-professional collaboration to ensure adequate discharge planning. It is acknowledged that boundaries often need to be extended and professional barriers dismantled (McClelland, 1985).

The maintenance of any successful programme of discharge planning requires an organisational commitment (Rasmusen and Buckwalter, 1985). Research both in the UK (Harding and Modell, 1989) and in the US has shown that inadequate discharge planning can lead to an increased readmission rate (Schrager et al., 1978). This is of concern not only to a diagnosis related group (DRG) system of costing health care but to any system striving to become more cost-effective and provide quality patient care. There are, however, inevitable cost implications in the provision of an effective health care continuum and a verbal commitment to discharge planning needs to be reflected in an appropriate allocation of resources.

The form that discharge planning arrangements may take is varied and a number of different approaches is described in later chapters. Reichelt and Newcomb (1980) stress the importance of *all* professionals having some responsibility for anticipating patients' needs after leaving hospital as a necessary condition for any discharge planning model to be effective.

The questions remain whether one person should have the major part, who this should be, and the extent to which clients are involved. The proposal that the hospital nurse should be responsible for a patient's discharge plan has an immediately attractive logic, especially if primary nursing is practised (Manthey, 1980), with accountability for an individual's total care resting with one nurse. It does, though, beg the question of how adequate a hospital nurse's knowledge of community services and care is when it comes to making an informed and realistic assessment. Without a clear and explicit assignment of discharge planning, the tendency is for it to be lost between a number of individuals.

Any form of discharge planning requires evaluation. Whether it is a named individual who makes referrals and coordinates communication, and whether that person is funded by hospital or community services, or whether the primary nurse or other hospital nurse is responsible for discharge planning arrangements, evaluation should be an ongoing process.

Client care outcomes are notoriously difficult to measure as it can be extremely difficult to isolate the variables and claim a causal relationship between nursing interventions in discharge planning and a patient's state of health and well-being. Muenchow and Carlson (1985) suggest that an individual discharge planning evaluation together with an overall programme evaluation are commonly present in the models they reviewed.

Until discharge planning is recognised as the responsibility of all health care staff in any setting and is seen as a common goal, then problems will remain. The onus currently placed on hospital staff to plan for discharge typically excludes community staff. The introduction of a liaison role may lift the burden of responsibility from hospital staff. Depending on how the liaison function is carried out, the hospital nurse may either perceive her role as having fewer responsibilities for discharge planning or take it as an opportunity which leads to a greater understanding of community care needs.

In the chapters that follow, the needs for planned discharge to effect continuity of care is acknowledged, from a variety of perspectives reflecting an author's particular interest in the subject. Each chapter is introduced by the editor to highlight key points. Margaret Macdonald (chapter 2) writes as a ward sister discharging patients to community care and Clare Newman (chapter 3) as a district nurse receiving patients referred. Bridie Fuentes (chapter 4.2) describes her work as a paediatric liaison health visitor and Felicity Watson (chapter 7) the evolution of a scheme within which the liaison role changed over time. Jan O'Leary (chapter 4.1), who currently manages a liaison team in West Suffolk, and Roger Deeks (chapter 5), with management responsibilities for a community hospital in Wales, describe from very different perspectives how liaison works for them. The research study described by Denise Barnett (chapter 8) used nursing process evaluation as a communication link between hospital and community . Sarah Jowett and Sue Armitage (chapter 6) tackle the concept of liaison and what it means to nurses, describing the first two years of an evaluation study of the liaison role. Finally, the perspective of patients is examined by Sue Armitage (chapter 9) as a component of the second two-year action research phase of the evaluation study on liaison in which hospital and community nurses met together on a regular basis to effect change.

Continuity of patient care is acknowledged as important to patients and staff in the quality of care received and given. It is easy to give lip service to it but difficult to achieve. In the chapters that follow the period of transition falling wholly into neither 'hospital' nor 'community' is examined. The intention is to point to a central focus for future action.

## References

Age Concern (1975) *Going Home.* Liverpool: Age Concern.

Amos G (1973) Age Concern Continuing Care Project *Care is Rare.* Liverpool: Age Concern.

Armitage S K (1979) *Interaction processes affecting the social diagnosis and referral of medical in-patients.* Newcastle upon Tyne Polytechnic: CNAA.

Armitage S K (1981) Negotiating the discharge of medical patients. *Journal of Advanced Nursing* **6**, 385–9.

Armitage S K (1989) Liaison nurse: the key to continuity of care. In *Good Practices in Community Nursing*, Monograph No.2. University of Manchester, Department of Nursing.

Bradshaw J (1972) A taxonomy of social need. In G McLachlan (ed.) *Problems and Progress in Medical Care,* seventh series. Oxford: Oxford University Press for the Nuffield Provincial Hospitals Trust.

Buckwalter K C (1985) Exploring the process of discharge planning: application to the construct of health. In McClelland, Kelly and Buckwalter (eds) *Continuity of Care: Advancing the concept of discharge planning.* London: Grune & Stratton.

Cass S K (1978) The effects of the referral process on hospital in-patients. *Journal of Advanced Nursing* **3**, 563–9.

Chaplin N (1982) *Getting it Right? The 1982 reorganisation of the National*

*Health Service*. London: The Institute of Health Service Administrators, second edition, Management Series 3.

Dartington T (1974) Fragmentation and integration in health care: the referral process and social brokerage. *Sociology of Health and Illness* **1**, 1, 12–39.

DHSS (1972) *Management Arrangements for the Reorganised Health Service*. London: HMSO.

DHSS (1986a) *Neighbourhood Nursing – a focus for care* (Cumberlege Report). London: HMSO.

DHSS (1986b) *Nursing Care in the Community – An initial study*, Vol. 1. Report of the Joint Management Study of the Community Nursing Services, Chair D V Hayward. Northern Ireland: DHSS.

DHSS (1987) *Promoting better health*, Cmd 249, *The Government's Programme for Improving Primary Health Care*. London: HMSO.

Department of Health (1989) *Discharge of Patients from Hospital* (with Health Circular HC(89)5).

Draper P (1986) Any use for an American import? *Nursing Times* **82**, 2, 37–9.

Edwards N (1987) *Nursing in the community – A Team Approach for Wales*. Review of community nursing in Wales (Chairman Noreen Edwards). Cardiff: Welsh Office.

Garret G (1985) Sharing the caring: the hospital and community in care of the elderly. *The Professional Nurse* **1**, 1, 19–22.

Gilchrist B (1987) Discharge planning: a priority for nurses? *Geriatric Nursing and Home Care* **7**, 12, 16–18.

Griffiths R (1988) *Community Care: Agenda for action*, A report to the Secretary of State for Social Services by Sir Roy Griffiths. London: HMSO.

Harding J and Modell M (1989) Elderly people's experiences of discharge from hospital. *Journal of the Royal College of General Practitioners* **39**, 318, 17–20.

HC(89)5 (1989) *Discharge of patients from hospital*. London: Department of Health.

Hockey L (1968) *Care in the Balance*. London: Queens Institute of District Nursing.

Jowett S A and Armitage S K (1988) Hospital and community liaison links in nursing: the role of the liaison nurse. *Journal of Advanced Nursing* **13**, 5, 579–87.

LAC(89)7 (1989) *Discharge of Patients from Hospital*. London: Department of Health.

Luker K A (1988) Do models work? *Nursing Times* **84**, 5, 27–9.

Mageean R J (1986) Study of 'discharge communications' from hospital. *British Medical Journal* **293**, 6557, 1283–4.

Manthey M (1980) *The Practice of Primary Nursing*. Boston: Basil Blackwell.

McClelland E, Kelly K and Buckwalter K C (eds) (1985) *Continuity of Care: Advancing the concept of discharge planning*. London: Grune & Stratton.

McClelland E (1985) National and international comparisons of continuity of care. In McClelland, Kelly and Buckwalter, *Continuity of Care, op. cit.*

McKeehan K M (ed.) (1981) *Continuing Care. A multidisciplinary approach to discharge planning*. St Louis: C V Mosby.

Melia K M and Macmillan M S (1983) *Nurses and the Elderly in Hospital and the Community: A study of communication*, Report prepared for the Scottish Home and Health Department, Nursing Research Unit, University of Edinburgh.

Muenchow J D and Carlson B B (1985) Evaluating programs of discharge planning. In McClelland, Kelly and Buckwalter, *Continuity of Care, op. cit.*

Nicklin P (1984) Innovation without change. *Senior Nurse* **1**, 3, 9–10.

*Nursing Standard* (1988) 'Cumberlege update' **2**, 23 April, 29.

Reichelt P A and Newcomb J (1980) Organizational factors in discharge planning. *The Journal of Nursing Administration* **10**, December, 36–42.

Rasmusen L A and Buckwalter K C (1985) Discharge planning in acute care settings: an administrative perspective. In McClelland, Kelly and Buckwalter, *Continuity of Care op. cit.*

Richmond M E (1917) *Social Diagnosis*. Russell Sage Foundation.

Roberts I (1975) *Discharged from Hospital*. London: Royal College of Nursing.

Schrager J *et al.* (1978) Impediments to the course and effectiveness of discharge planning. *Social Work in Health Care* **4**, 1, 65–7.

Skeet M (1970) *Home from Hospital: A study of the home care needs of recently discharged hospital patients*, 4th edition. London: Macmillan Journals.

Skeet M (1980) *Discharge Procedures – practical guidelines for nurses*. London: Macmillan.

Skeet M (1982) *Home from Hospital: providing continuing care for elderly people. Some key issues and learning experiences from the field.* Birmingham: King's Fund Centre.

Simpson J E P and Levitt R (1981) *Going Home. A guide for helping the patient on leaving hospital.* Edinburgh: Churchill Livingstone.

Slack G and Gibbins J (1979) *Organising Aftercare.*London: Continuing Care Project, National Corporation for the Care of Old People.

Thurstans J (1980) *Home from Hospital – to what?* Birmingham: Continuing Care Project.

UKCC (1987) *Project 2000: A new preparation for practice*. London: UKCC.

Webb C (1984) On the eighth day God created the nursing process and nobody rested. *Senior Nurse* **1**, 33, 22–5.

WHC(89)23 (1989) *Nursing in the community: A team approach for Wales*. Cardiff: Welsh Office.

Wright S G (1985a) How one nurse was converted. *Nursing Times* **81**, 33, 24–7.

Wright S G (1985b) It's all right in theory. . . . *Nursing Times*, **81**, 34, 19–20.

Wright S G (1986) A plea for plain English. *Senior Nurse* **5**, 4, 5.

# 2
# Slaying Snakes and Building Ladders: Transferring Patients Home

### Margaret Macdonald

## EDITOR'S INTRODUCTION

The difference between a community nurse's account of the transfer of patient care and a hospital nurse's is obvious: a community nurse cares for the patient after he has left hospital and the event of discharge is behind him; a hospital nurse is dealing with the potential, the planning for what might happen or for what it is hoped and anticipated will happen.

In this chapter Margaret Macdonald closely examines the role of the ward sister in planning an effective transfer of patient care. Central to the discussion is the acknowledgement of the boundaries of the experience of hospital nurses.

A detailed strategy for action is proposed for the development of necessary skills and experience for nurses within an overall, defined statement of beliefs. The importance of making baseline assessments against which future measurements of achievements can be made is stressed. For this to be effective the role of the ward sister as leader of a coherent team which discusses a shared commitment to care is emphasised. At the same time as facilitating her nursing team in their learning, the ward sister is required to involve them in the developing strategy and ensure their commitment to it.

The ward sister's role is regarded as pivotal and a challenging list of attributes is outlined as essential in enabling her to take up and carry through the responsibilities, thereby ensuring that effective continuity of patient care can take place. The ward sister is seen as requiring an understanding and clear concept of her role, not solely within a nursing framework but beyond that to other disciplines within and outside the hospital on an equal and reciprocal basis.

This is not a once-and-for-all campaign. Against the backdrop of educational and managerial support it is proposed that the ward sister should wage a continuous strategy of action in order to ensure adequate continuity of care for all patients.

## THE TRANSFER GAME

As a learner nurse, transferring patients home from hospital always seemed like an enormous and deadly game of snakes and ladders, in which the fate of individual patients and the continuity of their care rested upon the toss of a die. When I became a staff nurse, although there still appeared to be a preponderance of snakes and a paucity of ladders, I acquired skills in avoiding the former and seeking out the latter. On promotion to ward sister, however, it was evident that this was not sufficient. The time had come to consider slaying snakes and building ladders. This chapter outlines:

- the current state of play on the snakes and ladders board,
- the achievements which may be sought by the ward sister in the snake-slaying/ladder-building campaign,
- the assessing, planning, waging and evaluation of that campaign,
- the armour, equipment and support required by the ward sister involved in such activities.

In other words, after a brief discussion of the *issues* surrounding continuity of care, the role of the ward sister and the nursing team in transferring patients home will be discussed in terms of the *outcomes* to be achieved, the *process* undertaken and the *structure* required.

## THE ISSUES: THE CURRENT STATE OF PLAY

For the ward sister intent on slaying snakes and building ladders, the first priority must be to identify the issues to be confronted.

It may have been tempting in years gone by for the ward sister and the nursing team to view the transfer of patients home from hospital as an event discrete from other aspects of ward nursing practice. It may equally have been alluring to consider transfer planning as an isolated activity targeted at the occasional, usually elderly patient who, on leaving hospital, required the services of the community nursing staff. It has long been acknowledged that such transfers of care were often characterised by the inadequacy or inaccuracy of referral, but were seen to call for more detailed discharge documentation or more elaborate hospital–home liaison schemes. Thus, while matters of documentation and of liaison have been repeatedly examined and addressed, ward nursing practices have been preserved which permit snakes to flourish and ladders to crumble and decay.

Such a stance, however, is becoming increasingly untenable. Discharge or transfer has been defined as 'a stage in patient care situated towards one end of a continuum which has both a period of preparation and from which there are consequences' (Armitage, 1981).

If this definition is accepted, it is difficult for the ward sister and the nursing team to ignore the possibility and probability that the quality of a patient's aftercare stems, in part, from the quality of ward nursing practice. When transfer planning is seen to be required by all patients leaving hospital – whether the transfer of health care responsibilities is to the patient, the family and friends, or to the community-based voluntary and statutory services – then the scale of the challenge to the ward sister becomes apparent.

Research studies, moreover, clearly indicate aspects of ward nursing practice which contribute to the discontinuity of care between hospital and home (Hockey, 1968; Skeet, 1970; Roberts, 1975). It is demonstrated that hospital staff, in transferring health care responsibilities, repeatedly fail to communicate adequately, accurately and appropriately with the patient, family and friends, or the community-based voluntary and statutory services.

These identified shortcomings in ward nursing practice are believed to reflect other fundamental problems, including:

- attitudes and values among ward nursing staff, which militate against the patient being treated as an individual, the individual as part of a family, and the family as integral to the community;
- the emphasis in basic and continuing education on hospital, as opposed to community, nursing;
- ambiguous accountability at ward level for transfer planning and associated decision-making;
- the fragmented pattern of ward communication.

As the issues surrounding continuity of care embrace the quality of communication with patients, families, community and hospital colleagues as well as accountability for care, the preparation and development of nurses, and attitudes and values held by clinical staff, it would seem that there are major implications for the nursing profession in general and for the ward sister and ward nursing practice in particular. It could, indeed, be argued that the quality of the transfer home from hospital constitutes a performance indicator of ward nursing practice and of ward sister achievement. This examination of the current state of play, therefore, not only outlines the relationship between transfer home and ward nursing practice, but also indicates snakes that may be slain and ladders that may be built.

## OUTCOMES: THE ACHIEVEMENTS SOUGHT BY THE WARD SISTER

The next item on the ward sister's battle plan is, in conjunction with the nursing team, to draw up a statement of aims. It may seem a little unusual at such an early stage to be discussing what it is the ward sister is striving for in her snake-slaying/ladder-building campaign. There can, however, be little doubt that it is vital for the ward sister to have from the outset a clear concept of what she intends to achieve.

The aims or outcomes of the campaign are, for the most part, inherent in the recommendations of research studies on the subject of discharge home from hospital (Hockey, 1968; Skeet, 1970; Roberts, 1975). Retrieved and rephrased, the outcomes sought appear to be threefold. At the time of transfer home from hospital:

1. the patient will be as informed, independent and in control of care as individual circumstances permit;
2. the family and/or friends will be competent and confident to render any necessary assistance or support;
3. the community services (statutory and voluntary) will be appropriately and adequately involved in giving or supplementing care.

Such a statement of aims or outcomes provides the ward sister and the nursing team with a direction for their activities and a focus for their campaign of innovation in ward nursing practice.

## PROCESS: ASSESSING, PLANNING, WAGING AND EVALUATING THE CAMPAIGN

Rather than embarking rashly on an orgy of snake-slaying and a frenzy of do-it-yourself ladder construction, the ward sister and the nursing team need to:

- assess where ward nursing practice is in relation to the statement of outcomes;
- plan strategies to meet any shortfall identified in the assessment phase;
- implement these strategies;
- critically evaluate their effectiveness against the outcomes stated above.

At each stage in this campaign there is a variety of ways in which research findings may be applied to ensure more informed ward nursing practice in the future.

## The Assessment Phase of the Campaign

Although ward nursing practice in terms of transferring patients home from hospital has already been briefly discussed in general terms, each ward sister and nursing team will want to assess in greater detail the situation in their own clinical area. The nature of the campaign, after all, will vary according to the client group served, the medical specialty, the rate of patient turnover, nurse staffing levels and skill-mix, the education and training profiles of staff, communication systems, patterns of care, and staff attitudes and values. Several methods may be employed to determine where current ward nursing practice stands in relation to the statement of outcomes. These include the use of a recognised quality of care evaluation tool, and the application of relevant research findings in a comparative review of ward nursing practice. Both of these possibilities will be considered in detail as assessment forms the basis for planning, waging and evaluating the campaign.

As transferring patients home from hospital raises many issues fundamental to nursing care, the ward sister may consider it appropriate to make a baseline assessment of ward nursing practice by using a recognised quality of care evaluation tool. Should this be so, most health authorities have a designated person with responsibility for quality assurance whom the ward sister may contact for advice on the local availability and application of such instruments. Although communication with patients, relatives and the community services is not the exclusive focus of the tools, these aspects of care are touched upon to a greater or lesser extent within each. Initial assessment of the patient's physical and psychosocial needs, the planning of nursing care to meet these and the implementation of patient and family teaching are among the relevant criteria examined in *Monitor* (Goldstone et al., 1983). While the quality of the nurse-patient relationship is explored by the *Quality Patient Care Scale* (Wandelt and Ager, 1974), ward nursing practice is evaluated in terms of the skills of the individual practitioners in the *Slater Nursing Competences Rating Scale* (Wandelt and Stewart, 1975). If available and applied, any of these instruments may provide a relatively objective, if non-specific, measure of ward nursing practice.

Alternatively, or additionally, the ward sister and the nursing team may look to the research findings of studies on communication with patients, with relatives and with the community services. These offer numerous examples of good nursing practice and of barriers to such practice. Much of this information may be extracted and employed for the purposes of comparison with existing practice. The possibility of becoming submerged in, and ultimately swamped by, the volume of relevant data is very real. For this reason, only a very small sample of the pertinent research or research-based literature will be cited. While merely providing an insight or overview, these articles incorporate references for further exploration and study if required.

Studies on communication with patients clearly demonstrate that, on many occasions, information-giving, patient teaching and counselling are important keys to fostering patient control and independence (Wilson-Barnett, 1983; Price, 1984; Boyd, 1987; Close, 1988, Wilson-Barnett, 1988). The studies propose theoretical frameworks within which nurse-patient communication may be developed and documented. Examples of good practice in preparing patients for diagnostic and therapeutic procedures are also provided and in education or counselling of diagnosis related groups, such as patients with diabetes mellitus, myocardial infarction or the various forms of cancer. More specifically, good practice in terms of pre-discharge teaching to encourage, for example, independence in self-medication on discharge, is described (Clay and Stirn, 1986; Wade and Bowling, 1986; Markey and Igou, 1987). In summary, these studies outline the how, when, why and where of communicating with patients.

There is convincing evidence within the same works, however, that nurses repeatedly fail to employ information-giving, patient teaching and counselling strategies. Numerous reasons for this phenomenon are suggested. In the first place, nurses may not be able to differentiate between the various strategies, nor fully understand the correct application of each. They may not perceive themselves, nor indeed be perceived by others, as appropriate sources of information. With some justification, nurses may not believe that basic and post-basic education has equipped them with the knowledge, skills and attitudes to teach and counsel patients. Other nursing work, particularly the implementation of physical care, is observed to take precedence over psychosocial aspects of nursing practice. Patterns of organising patient care, moreover, may not always foster the continuity of care which enables teaching and counselling to occur effectively. In brief, many nurses do not appear to consider themselves accountable for their communication with patients.

Similarly, there is an increasing volume of research-based literature advocating not only information-giving, education and counselling of relatives, but also their appropriate involvement in care throughout the patient's hospital stay (Hawker, 1982; Darbyshire, 1987b; Davies, 1987). These aspects of ward nursing practice are seen to be important both because the greatest proportion of aftercare or assistance with aftercare is given by relatives or significant others (Hockey, 1968; Waters, 1987b) and because informed support from family and friends contributes to patient recovery (Webb and Wilson-Barnett,

1983; Webb, 1986). The need for sufficiently flexible visiting patterns to meet individual patient and family requirements and to facilitate communication and relative involvement in care is emphasised.

Yet again, there is substantial evidence that meaningful communication with, and significant involvement of, relatives and friends does not always occur. By providing an analysis of nurse-relative interaction in the hospital setting, one study highlights this discrepancy between theory and practice (Hawker, 1982). Of all nurse-relative interactions within this study, 75 per cent are observed to be initiated by relatives. The very real difficulties experienced by relatives in accomplishing this seemingly simple task are outlined. First, the relative must make the decision in principle to interrupt a nurse, before setting out to find one who appears to be 'interruptable'. The nurses, describing relatives as an intrusion into their flow of work, are seen to employ a variety of avoidance tactics, such as adopting 'a legitimate gait' or 'seeing but not seeing' the relative. When 'hovering' and other 'intention displays' have failed to attract and hold the nurse's attention, relatives are observed, on occasions, to abandon altogether their quest for dialogue. This study and others suggest again that many nurses may not believe themselves to be accountable for this aspect of ward nursing practice.

The importance of effective communication between ward nursing staff and the community voluntary and statutory services has, for decades, been vociferously discussed (Hockey, 1968; Skeet, 1970; Roberts, 1975; Bowling and Betts, 1984a and b; Moss, 1986; Barnett, 1986; Gilchrist, 1987). In order to increase awareness of community resources, the literature advocates the availability to nurses of comprehensive information about local community services. Establishing professional development programmes which permit ward nurses the opportunity of working alongside their community colleagues is also thought to facilitate smoother hospital-home transition. Examples of tried-and-tested transfer checklists and discharge documentation abound (Moss, 1986; Barnett, 1986; Gilchrist, 1987; Mezzanotte, 1987). Shorter communication channels are recommended, either by ensuring direct ward sister-community nurse contact, or by adopting variations on the community liaison nurse theme. The seeking of feedback – either positive or negative – from community agencies about each referral is considered likely to promote more constructive hospital-community relations. Research-based literature on communications with community services, therefore, offers the ward sister pointers to good ward nursing practice in this area.

Despite this expenditure of literary energy, many articles on transition from hospital to home still read like catalogues of disaster.

Insufficient knowledge on the part of ward nurses about community resources, inability to identify those at risk on transfer, poor oral and written communication skills and inadequate feedback to ward nursing staff about the quality of transfer of health care responsibilities have all been shown to contribute to this unsatisfactory situation (Bowling and Betts, 1984a and b; Moss, 1986; Waters, 1987 a and b).

Following such a review of relevant literature, the ward sister and the nursing team have a more detailed understanding of aspects of their ward nursing practice which may inhibit or enhance communication with patients, their families and the various community agencies. They have, in other words, a much clearer concept of the snakes and ladders of transferring patients home from their hospital ward. With these in mind, the ward sister, by discussion with patients, relatives and staff, by observation of ward activities and nursing behaviour, by reviewing nursing records and by inviting peer comment, may make an assessment of where nursing practice in the particular clinical area stands in relation to the statement of aims or outcomes.

The ward sister may, for example, ask patients about their satisfaction or dissatisfaction with information given to them. In doing so she is aware that patients usually express high levels of satisfaction with nursing care and thus treats these data with caution. The ward sister may also canvas relatives about the quality of information they have received. Nurses' views may be requested on their preparation and accountability for patient teaching, and on their commitment to involving relatives appropriately in patient care. Community nurse feedback on specific transfers may be sought. Interactions between nurses and relatives may be discreetly observed and the ward's visiting policy scrutinised. Nursing records may be scanned for evidence of documented patient teaching or signs of systematic and timely transfer planning. The ward's teaching programme may be examined to check if the importance of communication and continuity of care is reflected within it. To ensure a measure of objectivity, the ward sister may wish to utilise peer review by inviting an experienced practising nurse from hospital or community to help in this assessment.

During the assessment phase, therefore, the ward sister and the nursing team, in an attempt to ascertain where nursing practice stands in relation to stated outcomes, may either employ a recognised quality of care evaluation tool to provide an objective, non-specific measure of care, and/or apply criteria from research studies to give a more subjective, but more specific, evaluation of ward nursing practice. This baseline assessment may then be documented for future reference.

## The Planning Phase of the Campaign

The ward sister and the nursing team are now ready to progress to the second phase of the campaign. This involves the planning of strategies to meet any shortfall identified in the assessment phase between ward nursing practice and the statement of aims. A number of factors may affect the strategy options.

In the first instance, not all aspects of practice relating to continuity of care between hospital and home fall within the ward sister's remit. It is, after all, the doctor, who, on the vast majority of occasions, pronounces the patient medically fit for discharge, although the ward sister and, indeed, the patient, may negotiate the actual transfer date. While the organisation of nursing care is clearly within the ward sister's authority, she cannot control, but merely influence, the quality of communication within the ward's multidisciplinary team. A radical change of emphasis in basic and post-basic education is evidently beyond the power of the ward sister to advocate or achieve. She may, however, in collaboration with the School of Nursing staff, effect a shift of focus in the ward teaching programme and in the development of the staff nurses. It may be important, therefore, in the second phase of the campaign, for the ward sister to acknowledge and differentiate between the scope of her authority and the extent of her influence.

Secondly, the selection of campaign strategies will take into account the fact that the ward sister does not work 24 hours a day, 7 days a week, 52 weeks a year. As a ward manager, the important issue is not what happens when the ward sister is there, but what happens when she is not (Blanchard and Lorber, 1984). This being so, the ward sister will set out to build ladders that do not require her constant, stabilising presence at their base to keep them in position.

Although strategy details may vary according to assessment findings, common outline strategies may be identified by returning to the fundamental issues of nursing practice which underlie communication deficits. These include:

- attitudes and values of ward nursing staff;
- the focus of education and professional development;
- ambiguous accountability for transfer planning;
- fragmented patterns of ward communication.

An outline strategy to address each of these may be developed. The ward sister and the nursing team may, therefore, opt to:

- write or rewrite the philosophy for ward nursing practice;
- design or redesign the ward-based staff development programme to reflect that philosophy;
- organise or reorganise nursing care to ensure accountability for holistic patient care;
- structure or restructure communications within the ward team.

To these four outline strategies, details of focus and emphasis may be added and a tentative timescale for their achievement set.

## Waging the Campaign

A philosophy for ward nursing practice, a ward-based staff development programme, the organisation of nursing care and a framework for ward communications may all contribute to achieving continuity of care on transfer home.

### A Philosophy for Ward Nursing Practice

At the outset there are a number of questions that nursing staff may wish to ask the ward sister. What is a philosophy for ward nursing practice? Who should be involved in its creation? Why bother with one? How may such a philosophy affect the quality of a patient's transfer home from hospital?

First, then, what is a philosophy for ward nursing practice? A philosophy in this context has come to mean, quite simply, a statement of the nurses' beliefs and values about the patient, his family and friends, and the care, education and support they should receive in the ward. It may also include a statement of the nursing staff's beliefs and values about the qualified nurse, the learner and nursing auxiliary, and the place of each of these within the nursing team and the ward's multidisciplinary team.

Who should be involved in the drawing up and reviewing of such a statement? It is absolutely essential that the philosophy be drafted by, and meaningful to, all members of the ward nursing team. It may be tempting for the ward sister to settle herself comfortably in the confines of her office and compose an eloquent, sophisticated statement. She has, after all, explored the issues of continuity of care, identified the aims of the campaign, assessed ward nursing practice and selected strategies for change. Such a unilateral declaration of beliefs and values might, at best, be learned by rote and recited as ritual, and, at worst, be destined for obscurity on a dusty duty-room shelf. If, on the other hand, the ward sister has included the nurses at all stages of the snake-slaying/ladder-building campaign, then their involvement in writing this philosophy document is a natural progression from this. In order that the statement may reflect developing practice and the values of newly appointed staff, it is important to review the philosophy at regular, perhaps six-monthly, intervals. Written and reviewed in this way, the philosophy will be a dynamic, rather than a static, statement, belonging to, but not foisted upon, the nursing team.

Why should the nursing team expend time, energy and emotion on such a seemingly esoteric exercise? In the first instance, the drafting of a philosophy statement inevitably involves the nurses in a critical examination, not only of attitudes to patients, relatives and staff, but also of various aspects of nursing practice relevant to transferring patients home. Handled constructively, this may foster peer support, promote team spirit and a sense of common purpose. The drafting of a philosophy also permits the ward sister further insight into individual and group commitment to the aims of the campaign. The very process of writing a philosophy for ward nursing practice, therefore, serves a number of ends.

But how may the product of these deliberations, the completed philosophy statement, contribute to continuity of care on transfer home? It may be argued that a philosophy statement in which the nurses make an explicit commitment to the campaign aims and strategies is a prerequisite for innovation in ward nursing practice. A ward philosophy may, for example, state that the nurse:

- views the patient as an individual, the individual as part of a family, and the family as integral to the community;
- recognises the contribution of family and friends, who provide the majority of care and support before and after hospitalisation;
- includes the patient and, where appropriate, the relatives, in assessing, planning, implementing and evaluating care;
- offers the patient and relatives information, teaching and counselling appropriate to their needs and wishes;
- organises nursing care in such a way as to promote communication between the nurse, the patient and relative;
- acts as part of a wider team, which includes community-based staff and members of other health care disciplines within the hospital;
- endeavours to gain an understanding of the roles of these colleagues and to work and communicate constructively with them in the interests of continuity of care.

The implications of such a commitment are clear. For some nursing teams, however, these statements may go too far, for others not nearly far enough. Some practitioners may be ready to set written standards of care on such topics as patient teaching, relative involvement in care and transfer planning. Variations from ward to ward are inevitable. What is essential is that change in ward nursing practice is preceded by team commitment in principle to that change. The philosophy statement, therefore, serves not only as a measure of the nursing team's commitment to the aims and strategies of the campaign, but also as an indicator of the appropriate pace and degree of change.

One question remains. How can the ward sister and the nursing team translate the philosophy for ward nursing practice into a reality?

## A Staff Development Programme

One way of translating the philosophy into reality is to ensure that the importance of effective communication with patients, relatives and the community services is reflected within all ward-based education and development initiatives. This second strategy is discussed in relation to:

- the induction of newly appointed staff;
- continuing professional development of staff;
- the creation of a favourable environment for learner nurses.

Whether newly appointed nursing staff have had the benefit of a hospital orientation or induction programme or not, an introduction to the specific clinical area is essential. The content of this will depend on the nature of the particular ward and the needs of the individual nurse. In order that induction periods may contribute to the campaign aims, however, the ward-based programme may include:

- a discussion of the philosophy for ward nursing practice;
- an allocation of time with individual members of the multi-disciplinary team (the doctor, the medical social worker, physiotherapist, etc.);
- attendance at a multidisciplinary team meeting and a consultant ward round;
- an introduction to the ward's resource pack of local community services;
- a day with the community liaison nurse;
- an opportunity to work with a district nurse or health visitor;
- a session at the follow-up out patient clinic;
- a visit to ambulance control.

From the outset, therefore, the newly appointed nurse is aware of, and preparing for, the commitment to continuity of care between hospital and home.

Although there is an onus on the individual nurse to maintain and improve professional knowledge and competence, the ward sister has a responsibility to facilitate this process within the clinical area. Because of differing levels of clinical experience and diverse training and educational profiles, each ward nurse will require an individualised development programme. The ward sister may, however, compile a list or menu of essential and desirable objectives relevant to nursing care in the particular ward. This list or menu may emphasise the aims of the campaign by incorporating objectives relating to communication with patients, relatives and community colleagues. Each nurse, together with the ward sister, may then identify strengths and weaknesses and set personal objectives from the menu. Essential objectives for one nurse may, for example, include a statement that, at the end of a specified period of time, the nurse will be able to:

- assess, plan, implement and evaluate a teaching programme for a patient and relative;
- assess, plan, implement and evaluate, in partnership with the patient, family and community services, a plan of care for transfer home.

A desirable objective for a more experienced nurse may be to complete a counselling skills course. When this objective setting is linked with regular performance review, it may contribute substantially to meeting the continuity of care challenge.

The very fact that learner nurses have as mentors ward nurses committed to, and competent in, communication with patients, relatives and community colleagues, introduces the learners to the concept of continuity of care. The author has, moreover, found it useful to set imaginary case histories, from which the learners are required to plan transfers home from hospital. Copies of these scenarios are distributed to individual members of the multidisciplinary team, such as the community liaison nurse, the medical social workers and the ambulance controller. The learners then meet with each member of the multidisciplinary team in turn to discuss the completed discharge plans. These exercises not only assist learner nurses to develop discharge planning skills, but also promote communication between learner nurses and other health care professionals.

If the first strategy is about fostering a commitment to communication with patients, relatives and community colleagues, then the second strategy involves ensuring competence in these areas essential to continuity of care.

*Organisation of Nursing Care*

A third strategy available to the ward sister and the nursing team is to implement a method of organising nursing care, which is a suitable vehicle for the ward philosophy and the aims of the continuity of care campaign.

Some methods of organising care may be swiftly eliminated. Task allocation, for example, and even some interpretations of team nursing, are clearly at odds with a commitment to the patient and relative as individuals participating in care. The ward nursing team may, therefore, opt for one of the following:

*Team nursing*   in which each nurse has, during the span of duty, a specific allocation of patients within a team framework;
*Patient allocation*   in which each nurse is allocated a patient or group of patients for the span of duty;
*Primary nursing*   in which each patient is allocated a first level nurse to be accountable for her nursing care throughout the hospital admission.

But what evidence is there that evolution towards more patient-oriented approaches to organising care influences communications with patients, relatives and the community agencies?

A number of studies have demonstrated a significantly higher quality of care in primary nursing environments (Felton, 1975; Elpern, 1977; Eichhorn and Frevert, 1979; Steckel et al., 1980; Martin and Stewart, 1983). Of these, three studies report increases specifically in the quality of non-physical care (Eichhorn and Frevert, 1979; Steckel et al., 1980; Martin and Stewart, 1983). The founder of primary nursing, however, urges caution:

> Many people have mistakenly equated the concept of a system of care delivery with the concept of quality of care. The quality of nursing service in primary nursing can be good or bad, comprehensive or incomplete, co-ordinated or spasmodic, individualised or standardised, creative or routine. (Manthey, 1980)

It may be that patient allocation and, more particularly, primary nursing, while not guaranteeing a high quality of care, make absolutely clear the accountability for each patient's nursing care and its documentation. In other words, these methods of organising nursing care raise the visibility of the individual nurse's commitment to, and competence in, ward nursing practice relevant to continuity of care. This visibility enables the ward sister to adjust her management style and direct, coach, support or delegate to each member of her nursing team in an appropriate manner (Blanchard et al., 1985). If, for example, a nurse demonstrates a high level of commitment to the aims of the campaign but low competence in relevant practice, she will require supervision and direction from the ward sister. On the other hand, the ward sister may confidently delegate responsibility for day-to-day decision-making to the nurse who displays a high degree of both commitment and competence.

The decision to change the method of organising nursing care, requiring as it does a monumental shift in attitude and behaviour, is not to be taken lightly nor implemented overnight. It may be that the ward sister and the nursing team elect to move slowly and steadily along a continuum of change from, for example, team nursing to patient allocation and on to primary nursing. Thus, they gradually adopt a method of organising care which makes visible commitment to, and competence in, communication with patients, relatives and the community agencies. This permits the ward sister to manage her time and staff effectively and sensitively in the interests of continuity of care.

## A Framework for Communications Within the Ward Team

All the strategies of the ward nursing team to ensure effective information-giving, education and counselling will be to no avail unless the content of those communications is consistent with that which the patient, relative and community agencies receive from other health care workers. While, within the literature, there is evidence among health care professionals of a redefinition of roles, constructive and collaborative practice, and of shared learning experiences, there are also reports to the contrary. For some, multidisciplinary teamwork in the health care setting constitutes 'a myth' (Evers, 1981), or even 'a damaging development' (Appleyard and Maden, 1979). The doctor-nurse relationship has been compared to 'a transactional neurosis' (Stein, 1968) and their patterns of professional practice likened to 'the parallel play exhibited by toddlers' (Darbyshire, 1987a). Research studies into continuity or discontinuity of care between hospital and home, moreover, offer convincing testament to the fragmentation of communication among health care professionals. How can the ward sister and the nursing team, against this background, implement the fourth strategy of their snake-slaying/ladder-building campaign? In what ways can the nursing team contribute to the restructuring of ward communications?

In the exercise of her professional accountability, the nurse is expected to:

> Work in a collaborative and co-operative manner with other health care professionals and recognise and respect their particular contribution within the health care team. (UKCC, 1984)

By making a commitment to this clause of the UKCC *Code of Professional Conduct*, both within the ward philosophy and the initiatives of the staff development programme, the nursing team has laid the foundation upon which constructive dialogue with other health care professionals may be established. More than this is required, however. The ward sister and the nursing team must maximise existing opportunities and create new opportunities to develop that dialogue.

Existing opportunities for dialogue include the multidisciplinary team meeting and the multidisciplinary ward round. If, for example, the multidisciplinary team meeting is considered by nurses as an occasion to nod in hasty acquiescence to decisions taken, only to complain at length and at leisure, then there is enormous scope for change. By contributing frankly and assertively, the nurses may increase the likelihood that the multidisciplinary meeting may become an open and lively forum, where all options and opinions are explored before decision-making occurs. If the multidisciplinary ward round does not appear to involve the patient, the doctor, nurses and other health care professionals in a multilateral exchange of information, then there is room for improvement. With a little forethought, the nurses attending the ward round may identify and structure the information they intend to impart and the questions they plan to ask. The nurses may also help the patient and, where appropriate, relatives, before and during the ward round, by encouraging and assisting them to muster and, on occasion, present their information and questions. Following the ward round, the nurses may spend time with each patient to reiterate or expand upon information given, dispel misapprehensions and check that the patient is satisfied with the information exchanged and decisions reached. Opportunities for creating dialogue vary from ward to ward. The author, for example, has found that, if other health care staff are invited to participate in nursing induction and development programmes, then the nursing team may be asked to attend and take part in seminars and other events organised by the various health care professionals.

In these ways, the ward sister and the nursing team may contribute towards a restructuring of multidisciplinary communications within the ward, thus facilitating consistent communication with patients, relatives and community colleagues.

The implementation of the four campaign strategies may, therefore, significantly contribute to continuity of care between hospital and home. By writing a ward philosophy and designing a ward-based staff development programme, the ward sister and the nursing team may promote commitment to, and competence in, communicating with patients, relatives and community colleagues. A method of organising nursing care may be selected which makes that commitment and competence visible and permits these to be further developed. Fourthly, a restructuring of ward communications increases the likelihood that information received by patients, relatives and the community agencies will be consistent.

*The Evaluation Phase of the Campaign*

Finally, the ward sister and the nursing team will want to evaluate the success of the snake-slaying/ladder-building campaign. Such evaluation is an essential component of the campaign, rather than a last-minute addition or sudden afterthought. By meticulously identifying specific strategies and by performing a thorough baseline assessment of ward nursing practice, the nurses have paved the way for both formative and summative evaluation.

Formative evaluation comprises, quite simply, the regular monitoring of campaign progress. In planning the campaign, a tentative timescale for the achievement of the various strategies has been outlined. This permits the nursing team to chart progress on, for example, the drafting of the ward philosophy or the implementation of the staff development programme. Summative evaluation involves the nursing team, after perhaps a year, in repeating the original assessment of ward nursing practice using the same method(s). By comparing the results of the two assessments, the nursing team may identify areas of improvement, of minimal change or, indeed, of deterioration in practice. Unless this summative evaluation indicates full achievement of the campaign's aims, the ward sister may well find herself remustering the nursing team for a second campaign to tackle any surviving snakes!

## STRUCTURE: ARMOUR, EQUIPMENT AND SUPPORT FOR THE WARD SISTER

In order to assess, plan, implement and evaluate such a campaign, the ward sister requires a wide range of knowledge, skills and attitudes. These include:

- a belief that ward nursing practice may positively influence the quality of aftercare;
- a clear concept of the ward sister's role within and beyond the nursing team;
- an understanding of the scope of her authority and the extent of her influence;
- conceptual and problem-solving abilities;
- leadership qualities;
- expertise in the management of patient care, the management of people, resources and the process of change;
- skills in teaching staff and guiding their professional development;
- competence in the appreciation and application of research.

Is the ward sister adequately equipped and supported to take up the challenge of care continuity?

A cursory glance at the literature suggests that the ward sister is ideally placed to confront those problems of discontinuity between hospital and home arising from ward nursing practice. She is portrayed, after all, as the key figure in influencing standards of care, implementing change in nursing practice, in ward management and in the creation of a learning environment. Indeed, it has been said that the sister alone represents the continuity of social organisation to the patient and is forced to bridge the discontinuity of other people and services (Pembrey, 1980).

Closer scrutiny of relevant studies, however, indicates a number of general and specific problems which may impinge upon the effectiveness of ward sister interventions in this context. The ward sister is seen to experience a lack of clarity about her role within the nursing and multidisciplinary teams, and an uncertainty about the scope of her authority. These difficulties are compounded in some instances by inadequate preparation for the role and insufficient feedback on her professional performance. Also well-documented is the work and information overload of the ward sister, the fragmentation of her activities and communications and her non-management of nursing (Pembrey, 1980; Redfern, 1981, Runciman, 1983). More specifically, research demonstrates poor communication skills among ward sisters (Lelean, 1973), a lack of knowledge about how to mobilise community resources (Farnish, 1983), and the low priority placed by ward sisters on discharge planning (Roberts, 1975; Bowling and Betts 1984b; Waters, 1987a).

If such a campaign is to be undertaken, every effort must be made to provide the ward sister with pre-appointment preparation and post-appointment continuing education and development opportunities. These must include initiatives which promote the knowledge, skills and attitudes required to wage a snake-slaying/ladder-building campaign. It is, moreover, essential that the ward sister has a flexible and supportive management framework in which to function. By constructive dialogue and regular performance review, the ward sister and her senior nurse manager may move towards a shared perception of the ward sister role, the areas of a ward sister's control or influence, her objectives for achieving continuity of care, and the resources required. In other words, if the ward sister is to confront the issues of continuity of care, there are two prerequisites: educational support for the ward sister, and management support for the ward sister.

## CONCLUSION

In conclusion, therefore, discontinuity of care between hospital and home presents the ward sister, the nursing team and those who support the ward sister both educationally and managerially, with a challenge of quite heroic proportions. The ward sister and the nursing team have to acknowledge the relationship between ward nursing practice and the quality of a patient's aftercare, and recognise the enormous implications of that relationship. Aims for the campaign must be identified and ward nursing practice measured against these aims. Strategies that promote commitment to, and competence in, communicating with patients, relatives and the community agencies within a multidisciplinary framework must be planned, implemented and evaluated. The ward sister must be supported in her education and by management to enable all this to happen. In this way, the ward sister and the nursing team may set about the slaying of snakes, the building of ladders and the removal of all elements of chance or hazard from the process of transferring patients home from hospital.

## References

Appleyard J and Maden J G (1979) Multidisciplinary teams. *British Medical Journal* **2**, 6200, 1305–7.

Armitage S K (1981) Negotiating the discharge of medical patients. *Journal of Advanced Nursing* **6**, 5, 385–9.

Barnett D (1986) Smooth passage home. *Journal of District Nursing* **5**, 4–6.

Blanchard K and Lorber A (1984) *Putting the One Minute Manager to Work*. Glasgow: Collins.

Blanchard K, Zigarmi P and Zigarmi D (1985) *Leadership and the One Minute Manager*. Glasgow: Collins.

Bowling A and Betts G (1984a) Communication on discharge – 2. *Nursing Times* **80**, 32, 31–3.

Bowling A and Betts G (1984b) Communication on discharge – 5. *Nursing Times* **80**, 33, 44–6.

Boyd C W (1987) Patient education promotes transition from hospital to home. *Patient Education and Counselling* **9**, 3, 295–8.

Clay K L and Stirn M L (1986) Documentation of discharge teaching of patients who have had hip surgery. *Orthopaedic Nursing* **5**, 6, 22–4, 28.

Close A (1988) Patient education: a literature review. *Journal of Advanced Nursing* **13**, 2, 203–13.

Darbyshire P (1987a) The burden of history. *Nursing Times* **83**, 4, 32–4.

Darbyshire P (1987b) Sour grapes. *Nursing Times* **83**, 37, 23–5.

Davies J M (1987) Visiting acutely ill patients: a literature review. *Intensive Care Nursing* **2**, 4, 163–5.

Eichhorn M L and Frevert E I (1979) Evaluation of a primary nursing system using the Quality Patient Care scale. *The Journal of Nursing Administration* **9**, 10, 11–15.

Elpern E H (1977) Structural and organisational supports for primary nursing. *Nursing Clinics of North America* **12**, 2, 205–9.

Evers H K (1981) Multidisciplinary teams in geriatric wards: myth or reality? *Journal of Advanced Nursing* **6**, 205–14.

Farnish S (1983) *Ward Sister Preparation: A Survey in Three Districts*. Chelsea College, University of London: DHSS.

Felton G (1975) Increasing the quality of nursing care by introducing the concept of primary nursing. *Nursing Research* **24**, 1, 27–32.

Gilchrist B (1987) Discharge planning: a priority for nurses. *Geriatric Nursing and Home Care* **7**, 12, 16–18.

Goldstone L A, Ball J A and Collier M M (1983) *Monitor – An Index of the Quality of Nursing Care for Acute Medical and Surgical Wards*. Newcastle on Tyne Polytechnic Products.

Hawker R (1982) *The Interaction Between Nurses and Patients' Relatives*, unpublished doctoral thesis, University of Exeter.

Hockey L (1968) *Care in the Balance*. London: Queen's Institute of District Nursing.

Lelean S (1973) *Ready for Report, Nurse?* London: Royal College of Nursing.

Manthey M (1980) *The Practice of Primary Nursing*. Boston, MA: Blackwell Scientific.

Markey B T and Igou J F (1987) Medication discharge planning for the elderly. *Patient Education and Counselling* **9**, 3, 241–9.

Martin P J and Stewart A J (1983) Primary and non-primary nursing – evaluation by process criteria. *Australian Journal of Advanced Nursing* **1**, 1, 31–7.

Mezzanotte J (1987) A checklist for better discharge planning, *Nursing (US)* **17**, 10, 55.

Moss K (1986) Didn't I tell you? *Journal of District Nursing* **5**, 2, 4–6.

Pembrey S (1980) *The Ward Sister – Key to Nursing*. London: Royal College of Nursing.

Price B (1984) A framework for patient education, *Nursing Times* **80**, 32, 28–30.

Redfern S (1981) *Hospital Sisters*. London: Royal College of Nursing.

Roberts I (1975) *Discharged from Hospital*. London: Royal College of Nursing.

Runciman P J (1983) *Ward Sister at Work*. Edinburgh: Churchill Livingstone.

Skeet M (1970) *Home from Hospital*. London: Macmillan.

Steckel S B, Barnfather J and Owens M (1980) Implementing primary nursing within a research design. *Nursing Dimensions* **7**, 4, 78–81.

Stein L (1968) The doctor–nurse game. *American Journal of Nursing* **68**, 1, 101–5.

UKCC (1984) *Code of Professional Conduct for Nurses, Midwives and Health Visitors*. London: UKCC.

Wade B and Bowling A (1986) Appropriate use of drugs by elderly people. *Journal of Advanced*

*Nursing* **11**, 1, 47–55.

Wandelt M A and Ager J W (1974) *Quality Patient Care Scale*. New York: Appleton-Century-Crofts.

Wandelt M A and Stewart D S (1975) *Slater Nursing Competences Rating Scale*. New York: Appleton-Century-Crofts.

Waters K R (1987a) Discharge planning: an exploratory study of the process of discharge planning on geriatric wards. *Journal of Advanced Nursing* **12**, 1, 71–83.

Waters K R (1987b) Outcomes of discharge from hospital for elderly people. *Journal of Advanced Nursing* **12**, 3, 347–55.

Webb C (1986) Professional and lay social support for hysterectomy patients. *Journal of Advanced Nursing* **11**, 2, 167–77.

Webb C and Wilson-Barnett J (1983) Self-concept, social support and hysterectomy. *International Journal of Nursing Studies* **20**, 2, 97–107.

Wilson-Barnett J (ed.) (1983) *Recent Advances in Nursing – 6: Patient Teaching*. Edinburgh: Churchill Livingstone.

Wilson-Barnett J (1988) Patient teaching or patient counselling? *Journal of Advanced Nursing* **13**, 2, 215–222.

# 3
# Receiving Patients from Hospital
Clare Newman

## EDITOR'S INTRODUCTION

For most patients a hospital stay is an interlude in their lives. Normality means home. For many nurses whose focus of care remains with the institutional setting of a hospital, the reality of care is understandably within that hospital. District nurses who work in the community share the patient's perspective of hospital care as an interlude. For them, their hospital colleagues are a vital link for the continuity of care for patients returning home. As Clare Newman points out, discharge is not an outcome in itself but a stage along the systematic and individualised approach to continuing care when nursing process is fully undertaken. She discusses the importance of statutory and voluntary services working together to contribute to the continuity of care for patients who are no longer under the continuous observation of nurses as they are in hospital.

Drawing on a number of published reports concerned with community care, emphasis is given to the importance of working with colleagues from a number of disciplines.

Acknowledgement is made of the importance of the interrelationship of district nurses' work with others and their mutual understanding of each other's roles and contribution to continuity of patient care.

## PATIENTS, CARERS AND HEALTH

The popular image of the National Health Service is one in which acute hospitals and high technology predominate. Emergency care and pioneering treatments are accorded a high profile and little reference is made to the realities of health care across the spectrum.

We live in a time of changing demography and patterns of illness. The scourge of infection which accounted for so much morbidity and mortality in the past has given way to other health problems which tend to be more related to degenerative conditions and patterns of behaviour. Coronary heart disease, lung cancer and many accidents are prominent causes of death and disability and are in some way linked to lifestyle and therefore more amenable to eradication by education than by medical intervention. A rise in the number of people surviving to old age results in the prevalence of chronic and degenerative conditions such as arteriosclerosis, arthritis and dementia. The elderly are prey to multiple pathology which may limit the options for curative treatment. These circumstances point to an increasing need for health care along with cure, and for prevention of ill health by education and early detection. Meanwhile medical advances in diagnosis and treatment create expectations and ethical conflicts that change the meaning of health.

Regional and class inequalities in health (DHSS, 1980) and in health care provision and uptake persist. There is evidence that much ill health goes unreported and undiagnosed in the community (Williamson et al., 1964). Sociologists have demonstrated the subjectivity of interpretations of health, and that illness behaviour must be seen in its social context. The social context in which ill health and disability occur is changing. Families are smaller and geographically more mobile, and an increasing number of marriages end in divorce. Women's lives have altered: female paid employment outside the home is increasing. Unemployment and poverty have their own implications for health and for the support of dependants. It seems likely that a rising number of elderly people will be needing care from a shrinking and ageing pool of supporters.

In order for the health service to tackle the determinants of illness and to allow diagnosis, care and treatment to be accessible to those most in need, it is becoming clear that what is required is a greater emphasis on the primary health services, which are the first and often an individual's only point of contact with the NHS. A continuing drop in the average length of hospital stay, combined with the social changes already alluded to, is bound to have implications for community services in terms of the provision of direct care and of the need for more professional support for informal carers. In acknowledgement of the changing role of the district nurse, the new training curriculum is intended to prepare district nurses to 'take a positive approach to future developments to meet health care needs' (Panel of Assessors, 1978) and demands a study of sociology, psychology, epidemiology and social policy as well as preparation in teaching, communication, information gathering and management skills. Flexibility and the ability to adapt to change are the objectives of the United Kingdom Central Council in their Project 2000 proposals (UKCC, 1986) and a much greater commitment to learning in the community is envisaged.

Already an enormous amount of the care of ill and disabled people is carried out in the community. Although the elderly are heavy users of the health service, only approximately 5 per cent are in institutions at any one time (Hudson, 1984), a figure which may be at odds with commonly held perceptions of ageing and of geriatric care. The vast burden of nursing falls on informal and often untrained carers, and is difficult to quantify without the recourse to bed occupancy numbers which hospitals have at their disposal (Salvage, 1985). Currently 60 per cent of the health service budget is directed to hospital services, while 30 per cent is spent on community health and general practitioner services, although only 3 per cent of patients are treated on an in-patient basis (Hudson, 1984). Primary health care budgets are often not clearly delineated and therefore the impact of change on community nursing services, for instance, is difficult to assess (Edwards, 1987). Local authority budgets are unstable and none of the central government grant support is earmarked for expenditure on the elderly, mentally ill, mentally handicapped or physically disabled in the community (Griffiths, 1988). The result is often patchy service provision. Both health and social services authorities may sometimes be accused of a failure to acknowledge the contributions of the informal caring networks and work towards facilitating their efforts by providing coordinated care rather than poorly connected items of service.

Bonny (1984) found carers to be predominantly married women aged over fifty years. A substantial number were elderly themselves and many of the dependants were multiply handicapped. Tasks demanded of carers in the community range from basic personal activities such as washing, feeding and toileting, to more skilled procedures including injections, bronchial suction, catheter and stoma care and recording of blood pressure. The burden of the care often results not so much from the actual tasks involved (although these may be physically onerous or embarrassing) as from the unremitting nature of the commitment needed, the loss of privacy, freedom and social life, and from family conflict. Financial costs are not only direct, in terms of extra heating, laundry, transport and so on, but may be long-term, resulting from loss of work, promotion and pension rights. All these pressures can predispose to family breakdown and damage to the physical and mental health of the carer. Voluntary and statutory service provision for carers is not standard across authorities nor necessarily applied rationally to those most in need. Charlesworth et al., (1984) found, for example, variations in the home help and respite care provision offered to male and female carers.

Discharge from hospital is often a critical time in a person's life in terms of help required to make good a self-care deficit. Whether the hospital admission is in response to an acute event or a planned admission for cold surgery, the likelihood is that in many cases the individual will be less able to cope unaided at home, for a variable period, than prior to admission. Victor and Vetter (1984) found that following discharge from hospital, usage of health and social services by the elderly in the community increased markedly, and Waters' study (1987a) confirmed other findings that, for whatever reason, there is a trend after hospitalisation towards a lower level of independence in personal and domestic activities of daily living for the elderly. Physical needs in younger patients who have undergone, perhaps, planned surgery, are unlikely to be of the same order, and are generally compensated for by family members, but studies abound (Wilson-Barnett and Fordham, 1982) to suggest that the days or weeks following discharge from hospital can be fraught with anxiety and uncertainty about aftercare. There is evidence that for a variety of reasons the transfer of patients from hospital to community is not always well planned or executed.

## COORDINATION OF CARE, PAST AND PRESENT

Investigations into the process of hospital discharge have pointed up several recurring themes.

Planning for discharge has been, and sometimes remains, haphazard or non-existent. Skeet (1983) asserts that 'discharge from hospital should never come unexpectedly to a patient nor to those attending him', yet too often patients have received less than 24 hours' notice of their return home. Transport arrangements, home facilities, social and psychological preparations must often be inadequate in these circumstances. Waters (1987b) found that patient care plans rarely identified problems related to the return home, suggesting that discharge tends to be perceived as an end in itself rather than as a stage in a patient's career (Armitage, 1981).

A well-planned discharge will anticipate a patient's community needs, but shortfalls in the nursing, domestic and personal help offered to patients have repeatedly been found. Often, help with housework and shopping appears to be the most pressing need, but Skeet (1974) found 45 per cent of her respondents had unmet nursing needs, and that community services being used two weeks postdischarge were double those requested by hospital staff.

Underpinning many of the gaps in continuity of care are communication issues. Skeet (1974), Roberts (1975) and Waters (1987b) have all pointed up aspects of a communication block between hospital staff and their patients, particularly regarding advice on aftercare. Communication between hospital and community staff, too, is often poor and indirect. Roberts (1975) suggests that attitudes towards continuing care are more important in discharge than the actual procedures involved.

## DISCHARGE PLANNING

### Decision-making and the Multidisciplinary Team

The timing of a patient's discharge from hospital may be influenced by input from a multiplicity of sources and sometimes professional and patient expectations do not match. Hockey (1968) found that more patients considered themselves prematurely discharged than retained in hospital too long, while ward sisters tended to feel that they had patients in their care who no longer required hospital facilities. To tackle this lack of fit, the physical, social, psychological and environmental resources of a patient and family need to be considered prior to discharge, and for patients with complex needs the contributions of all members of the multidisciplinary team are essential. However, the sharing of information about a patient often appears to be inadequate. Waters (1987b) found hospital nursing documentation about patients markedly lacked detail but contained twice as much social information as did medical records. Yet in practice it is frequently medical staff whose opinion dictates the timing of discharge, and the clinical state of the patient may be considered to the exclusion of other essential factors. Pressure on bed space is inevitably a factor in the discharge of patients, as is the availability in the community for further care, for example day hospitals with physiotherapy amenities, 24-hour district nursing cover, availability of equipment. Returning patients to homes with inadequate social support or environmental facilities, or to carers lacking the necessary skills, knowledge or attitudes to cope, must in many cases be a prescription for repeated admission to hospital. It is essential that sound information from hospital and community nurses, doctors, social workers, occupational and physiotherapists, dietitians and others is pooled in order to make considered decisions about patient discharge. Nurses must be prepared and enabled to make known their knowledge of home circumstances detrimental to a patient's care. The history of nursing and its relationships with medical staff tend to militate against equal importance being attached to the contributions of all members, and nurses should be alert to being drawn into the 'doctor–nurse game' described by Stein (1967). Ingrained attitudes are difficult to break down, but the nurse should heed the challenge of the UKCC Code of Professional Conduct to 'ensure that no action or omission on his/her part or within his/her sphere of influence is detrimental to the condition or safety of patients/clients' (UKCC, 1984).

Central to the process of discharge is the patient of course, who may in turn contribute to the timing of discharge by overt negotiation or covertly by various delaying tacts (Armitage, 1981). In line with perceptions of the sick role (Parsons, 1951, cited in Bond and Bond, 1986), whereby the patient is expected to want to recover as quickly as possible and to cooperate fully in nursing care, professionals tend to see such negotiating behaviour as manipulative. All members of the nursing team need to be alert to veiled delaying strategies, and to have the necessary time and counselling skills to allow exploration of the patient's underlying anxieties.

## The Nursing Process as an Aid to Continuity of Care

The nursing process is a widely used tool, entailing a problem-solving approach to nursing. Important aspects are the emphasis on the individual, the holistic view taken, and the interaction with the patient. It offers a systematic means of assessing needs and planning, delivering and evaluating care.

Assessment provides a written comprehensive baseline account of a patient's position on a health–illness continuum, and takes account of the multiplicity of the influences on, and effects of, that position. Used in conjunction with a nursing model, the assessment directs attention to the patient as an individual, as part of a family, and as part of a wider social sphere, and places the patient in a temporal context: 'The process looks backwards to examine the antecedents of the patient needing care, it looks at the here and now . . . and it looks forward to the aftercare' (Ryland, 1981). Aside from the information gleaned, the benefits of the nurse/patient interaction involved in taking a nursing history include the involvement of the patient in nursing care, which may lead to increased compliance, the opportunities for nurses to help patients make informed choices, and a deeper commitment between patient and nurse. Nursing assumptions about what the patient sees as problematic may be enlightened. A proper assessment of patients in hospital will invariably demonstrate any needs which may have relevance to discharge, and regular review of these will ensure priorities and the direction of care are appropriate.

The planning part of the process inevitably involves nurses in justifying their choices of intervention, and thus in questioning routinised and non-research-based care. Again, the involvement of the patient is central. Focusing intervention on the attainment of patient-centred goals will prevent discharge from hospital being seen as an outcome in itself, and is particularly important in the care of chronically sick and disabled people whose care has in the past been lacking in specific direction (Kratz, 1978). Continuity of care should become a reality if this basis for nursing action is undertaken. Individual, undocumented nursing interpretations of the care required serve to work against a consistent approach and muddy the waters in building a body of knowledge on outcomes of nursing intervention. A detailed explicit plan is an important step in evaluating care.

The nursing process forces nurses to look at the means of care delivery and consider appropriate organisation of workload and use of skills. The process can be a useful tool for managers in deciding on resource allocation, particularly, in this context, staffing resources outside hospital. Data collected by nurses are often task-centred and little is learnt about effectiveness of care (Luker, 1983). The nursing process has much potential in determining efficacy and quality of care by examining goal achievement. There are difficulties associated with evaluation and demonstration of causal relationships between care and patient progress, particularly as measurement of concepts such as 'recovery' and 'dependence' are poorly developed (Wilson-Barnett, 1981) but over time it may become possible to be more predictive about outcomes.

However, there is a suggestion that the letter of the nursing process has been adopted to the exclusion of the spirit. 'When nurses claim that they are using the nursing process it is usually the beginning of the process which they have formalised, namely assessment' (Luker, 1983). Goals set are often inaccurate, unrealistic or unquantifiable, with the result that evaluation is impossible. Plans of care may be diffuse and open to interpretation by the various members of staff attending the patient, and may not fully take on board individual requirements. The introduction of the nursing process in some places has left much to be desired, and it is scarcely surprising that some nurses have viewed it as merely another exercise in paperwork, without understanding the contribution it can make to the continuity of care. Waters' study (1987b) showed that 80 per cent of identified problems remained unevaluated at the time of discharge, and that ongoing unresolved problems were not used as a basis of information in district nurse referrals.

## Discharge Preparation for Unresolved Problems

Discharge preparation, if it occurs at all, is sometimes a series of hasty procedures and not necessarily related to patients' real needs on return home. Nursing care needs to be directed, from admission onwards, to life outside hospital. Early mobilisation of patients from bedrest is generally accorded priority, but activities undertaken in hospital often bear little resemblance to those which will be part of everyday living at home. Few patients, for example, will be given the opportunity to dress themselves fully, climb stairs, lift a kettle, walk across a room crowded with furniture or reach a low electrical socket before discharge. Many patients are unprepared for the aches, pains, difficulties and fatigue associated with the first few days at home, and need to be warned to expect these in order to avoid uncertainty and anxiety. Patients' information needs are too often neglected. An indication of staff expectations of their recovery is often helpful. It is important to appreciate that verbal information given to people under stress will not always be assimilated and recalled. Nurses are discovering that advice on aftercare and recovery is not well retained by patients, or not elicited in the first place because patients regard their uncertainties as trivial or embarrassing (Vaughan and Taylor, 1988). The use of advice leaflets for discharged patients is increasing and is to be recommended, especially if they are individualised where necessary. Advice offered is often very negative, unspecific and incomplete (Wilson-Barnett and Fordham, 1982). To instruct a patient not to lift heavy weights, for instance, takes no account of the patient's perception of 'heavy' or 'lifting', nor of how long avoidance of lifting is expected: it is more important that the patient is taught proper lifting techniques and given an individual timescale over which to graduate exercise.

In view of estimates (Bliss, 1981) that 10 per cent of admissions to geriatric wards are due to iatrogenic disease, attempts must be made to ensure compliance with drug regimes on discharge, by teaching and *aides-mémoires*. Nurses have an important role in encouraging medical staff to simplify prescriptions as much as possible, and checking that medication is provided in an acceptable form. Wade and Bowling (1986) have reviewed some patient-education programmes on drug use. Community nurses can rarely undertake the administration of oral medication to patients: their role is to teach and supervise, but it is to be hoped that generally this will entail reinforcement of teaching that has taken place in hospital.

The psychosocial and environmental problems of patients need to be addressed early in a hospital stay and these will often require an interdisciplinary approach. Referral to or consultation with appropriate agencies may unnecessarily delay discharge if not undertaken soon enough. The enormous psychological difficulties associated with, for example, mutilating surgery or a diagnosis of life-threatening disease must be acknowledged and the patient and family given support outside the hospital. Patients whose needs on discharge clearly involve physical nursing are generally referred without any problem, but to ignore a patient's need for counselling and support can lead to much misery and ill health. In Anderson's study (1988) of mastectomy patients, concern was expressed about the low level of referral to community nurses where no nursing procedure was required.

Patients are sometimes less self-caring than they appear in hospital when left without round-the-clock supervision. Bearing in mind that district nurses can only be with patients for a fraction of the day, teaching must take account of possible contingencies, for example, hypoglycaemia or intercurrent illness for the diabetic. The patient's family has a vital part to play in adaptation and should therefore become involved in the learning process prior to discharge. Restricted visiting hours are not helpful to the smooth transition between hospital and home because they result in the loss of valuable opportunities for communication between the patient, carers and hospital staff. To give the impression that caring skills are the exclusive domain of trained nurses is to rob carers of their value and confidence in their capacity to cope, to the detriment of the rehabilitation of the whole family.

## Community Strengths and Limitations

When a patient's community needs have been assessed prior to discharge, the ward sister's knowledge of the national and local resources available to meet those needs is critical. Inevitably there will be local strengths and weaknesses. Allocating patients to the better known services without first determining needs may have the effect of diluting the evidence of unmet need, thus perpetuating any existing weaknesses. For example, the home help service is better manned in some areas than others and organisations such as the Crossroads Care Attendants scheme are not yet operating nationwide. There may be small extremely localised sources of financial aid such as clubs and guilds, employers may have well or poorly developed occupational health services, and so on. A sound knowledge of the networks of support available to patients in the community is seen as vital to community nurses (DHSS, 1986) but it is equally important for ward sisters if discharge is to be properly planned. Sometimes an attitude is encountered within statutory organisations that suggests the voluntary sector is unreliable, untrained and partisan, but it should be remembered that many of the statutory services were first tried out in the voluntary sector. Only by demolishing 'professional' barriers may the two sectors work together to ensure that the flexibility, experience and motivation of the one complements the accountability, education and overview of the other.

Local and national factors affecting the district nursing service must be appreciated by the ward sister in order that she may best utilise the service and make effective discharge plans. There may be, for instance, a clinic which the patient may attend for suture removal if the condition does not dictate a home visit. The level of provision during unsocial hours varies with health authorities. While some operate a 24-hour community nursing service, this is not always the case and may have implications for the care of the terminally ill patient in the community. Although the increasing use of syringe drivers and suppositories for narcotic analgesia may reduce the need for frequent injections in the final days of a patient's life, Cumberlege (DHSS, 1986) found a need for professional advice and support round the clock. In some authorities, however, it is felt that staff are more effectively concentrated during normal working hours during which their teaching and liaison capacity may best be exercised, and other means of meeting needs at night may be in operation, for example a Marie Curie service. Weekend nursing cover in the community is usually limited and may not work in a practice-attached way. Most hospital staff are aware that the 'Friday afternoon discharge' is not in the interest of the patient who needs extensive nursing or social services. Surgeries and pharmacies too tend to close outside normal working hours with the result that obtaining medication, dressings or equipment may be difficult. It is important that patients are provided with adequate supplies to last them until amenities are open. It is to be expected that, when district nurses are awarded prescribing powers, the rigours of obtaining dressings will become less great. District nurses are also faced with the perennial problem of the delay in availability on prescription of recent wound care products used in hospital. Many of the gels, foams and odour-reducing dressings may be impossible to acquire in the community, and ward sisters need to be aware of this limitation when selecting a dressing for a patient who is about to be discharged. Another problem may be the equipment necessary for the patient's care at home. Items such as commodes, pressure-relieving mattresses and nebulisers are often in great demand and it may be difficult for a discharged patient to acquire them without notice. It is generally possible to obtain equipment not available in stock from other sources such as the Red Cross, or to arrange funding by local voluntary bodies, but this obviously takes time to negotiate and should be considered when discharge plans are made.

## COMMUNICATION BETWEEN HOSPITAL AND COMMUNITY NURSES

### Attitudes to Community Care and Relationships between Colleagues

The esteem in which the district nursing service is held by hospital staff may be crucial in determining at what stage a patient is discharged home. Where personal contact between hospital and community staff is maintained, knowledge of each other's roles, capabilities and pressures is likely to be enhanced and this will help towards effective communication. However, in areas whose hospitals may serve large or ill-defined populations it may often be the case that no district nurse is on familiar terms with all sources of referral. Anonymity leads to the perception of stereotypes, and it is probably fair to say that the image held of district nurses by hospital staff may be rather rigid.

One stereotype of the district nurse is that she is primarily engaged in hygiene activities and the giving of tea and sympathy. This is the attitude which tends to foster 'task' referrals from hospital staff, often encouraging the patient to maintain contact with the ward for super-vision. Williams (1974) shows how the development of nursing as a profession rather than a vocation has led to the devaluation of basic intimate care and attachment of status to highly skilled technical pro-cedures. Hospitals are seen as the focus for these procedures and therefore bestow upon their workers the virtues of being more com-petent, more up-to-date, more 'professional'. What this image ignores, of course, is not only the fact that the district nurse is increas-ingly becoming involved in more technical aspects of nursing such as diagnostic procedures, care of patients on ventilators and enteral feeding, but also the importance of the psychosocial skills required to help patients and their families adapt to chronic disabling con-ditions, or to change their behaviour in order to prevent recurrence or aggravation of 'lifestyle' diseases.

Another image of the district nurse is that she is an experienced nurse possessed of an extra qualification, skilled in the assessment and care of patients in their own environments, whose work is fairly autonomous, and who would resent being given instructions on the care required by a patient. This stereotype tends to lead to referrals lacking any of the information which the district nurse needs in order to make a full assessment, perhaps through a wariness of 'treading on toes'.

This is not to deny that in many instances communication between ward and district nurses is satisfactory and sometimes excellent. Regrettably, much of the time, feedback to ward staff about the quality of discharge arrangements is limited, and good practice is therefore not rewarded. It would behove district nurses to make a habit of transmitting their appreciation to ward sisters who have made exhaustive preparations and communicated well. It is notable that a wide-ranging quality of discharging practice may be found within one unit whose procedures for communication are ostensibly standardised. Often, but not exclusively, these differences may be related to the category of patient and turnover of a ward, for example, acute surgical or elderly. The variations suggest that, however sound the system, it will only work well where continuity of care is valued by individuals and where knowledge of community issues is based on reality gleaned through experience. However, given these requisites, if systems are inadequate or confused, poor communication will often result: 'The virtue of method is the harness without which only the horses of genius travel' (Osler, 1975, cited in Stott, 1983).

### Routes of Communication

The very nature of district nursing means that the district nurse is inaccessible for communication with wards for much of her working day. Arrangements for referral vary in different areas but in general a telephone call is involved which frequently means messages being conveyed and distributed by receptionists or clerks. It is unrealistic to expect non-nursing personnel to be in a position always to transmit meaningful information about nursing care, and it is legendary that the essence and details of a message may become distorted as it is relayed by a number of people, however conscientious. District nurses need to examine the way in which their team's time is deployed in order to improve their availability for a dialogue with hospital staff, as well as with other agencies.

Telephoned messages may be preceded or followed by written communication about a patient. These are subject to the same delays as discharge letters to general practitioners. Studies showing unacceptable intervals between a patient's discharge and receipt by the GP of a summary letter are legion (Lefever, 1981; Neville, 1987; Harding, 1987), and Bowling and Betts (1984) found that referral slips to nursing staff could arrive 1–3 weeks after the patient's discharge giving information the nurse would have needed prior to visiting the patient. Giving the patient a discharge letter to hand to the district nurse on her first visit results in less delay, but may still not enable the nurse to be as prepared for the important initial visit as she would like to be. The problem inherent in this approach is that some nurses may feel certain kinds of information should not be transmitted by this means, such as when a patient for whatever reason is unaware of a poor prognosis.

### Documentation

The format of discharge letters to community nurses varies considerably from a brief letter-type document allowing space for biographical details and a few lines for free comment, to a highly structured form with heading and columns covering many aspects of a patient's care profile. The briefer 'letter' form probably requires less time to complete which must be a consideration for wards with a high patient turnover. Its unstructured nature may also allow for nursing staff to give a valuable 'thumbnail sketch' of a patient and the issues of principal concern and its personal tone of communication fosters a feeling of partnership in care. However, it does not encourage a systematic approach to giving information and almost inevitably leaves questions unanswered. One of the problems associated with the more structured type of discharge form is possibly the length of time it takes to complete properly. This, combined with the rigidity of its headings, may lead to a rushed approach which detracts from its potential as a rich source of information. Often this type of form tends to neglect the psychosocial aspects of a patient such as his reaction to his illness or operation, his knowledge of his diagnosis or prognosis, and what guidelines he has been given with regard to rehabilitation.

Hospital and community staff need to look closely at the possibility of shared documentation, particularly for use with patients with chronic problems whose life is likely to be interspersed with periodic hospital admissions. The use of the written care plan along the whole continuum of patient care could promote a vastly improved sharing of information between health professionals. Discharge summaries could at least be related to the format of the care plans in use in the area, with an emphasis on problems identified, care given and evaluated, and consideration given to the emotional and educational needs of the patient and his carers. Indeed, discharge summaries are only a part of the answer to closing gaps: transfer summaries may be used between hospital and community in both directions. Patient-held records or 'cooperation cards' are a valued feature of perinatal care, often used by more than one discipline, and there may be good reason to believe that this system of communication could be adapted and extended to other branches of patient care.

## Content of Information

One of the gifts with which district nurses may often wish they had been endowed is that of second sight! It is not unknown for the sum total of a hospital ward's communication regarding a patient's discharge to consist of a telephone message revealing the patient's name and address and the cryptic request to 'assess'.

The detailed nature of discharge information required will vary according to the individual patient, but in broad terms ward staff should consider information required for the first visit which will facilitate its timing, preparation and success as an assessment.

In an ideal world, anyone requiring a post-discharge visit from a district nurse would receive it within hours of arrival home but often in reality the district nurse needs certain information to allocate priorities. Insulin-dependent diabetics or the terminally ill, for example, may need a dose of insulin or analgesia at a specific time, and this should be conveyed clearly. For surgical patients it is not sufficient merely to give a date for removal of sutures: the nurse should know when the patient is to be discharged and the date of surgery in order to have some idea whether the patient requires interim visiting to monitor, among other things, recovery and pain control.

Another important factor in the timing of the first visit is the degree of social support the patient has and whether home assessment and adaptations have already been carried out by an occupational therapist. The district nurse is also particularly grateful if she is informed of any problems of access to the patient. It is helpful if she is made aware of any special needs the patient has for items of equipment which the hospital has been unable to supply in order that she may arrange for their availability or if necessary negotiate postponement of discharge in the event of their being unobtainable.

To maximise the effectiveness of the district nurse's assessment visit, information transmitted by ward staff should at least include a medical and nursing diagnosis, and any plans for future care envisaged such as attendance at day hospital facilities. Details of services provided by other agencies may be recalled only vaguely by patients and should be recorded to allow the district nurse to plan her care. Accuracy of information is often neglected; the size of a pressure sore or the actual reading of a blood pressure recording will give a baseline from which to work. The district nurse is not with her patient all day and cannot observe all that she needs to know about, for instance, a patient's mobility or pain or pattern of incontinence in the same way that these become clear over a period in hospital. Where a patient has communication difficulties, or where the use of patient- or carer-completed continence charts or pain diaries is inappropriate, it is helpful if as much detail is conveyed as possible. Information about the patient's knowledge and attitudes about his condition should be passed on, along with any specific aftercare advice given to the patient in order for the teaching to be reinforced. With an accurate picture of a patient's capacities and problems, care will not be given which promotes dependence unnecessarily or which fails to meet need.

## COMMUNICATION BETWEEN HOSPITAL AND PATIENT

District nurses too often find that, not only are they given inadequate information about patients, but that the patients themselves are in possession of very little knowledge about their illness, operation, treatment or aftercare. This lack is worrying in view of the evidence suggesting the importance of the role of information in preventing pain and anxiety.

For the patient to be an active participant in personal health decisions, rather than a passive recipient of professional judgement, nurses need to adopt the roles of facilitator, advocate, supporter and teacher. Patients entering hospital are subject to a culture of language, roles, routines and structures they may not begin to understand, at a time when the effects of their illness or disability are already enforcing adaptation. The interpersonal aspects of the nursing role are only recently beginning to receive their due attention, and many nurses feel insufficiently skilled, or organisationally enabled, to meet the patients' needs with regard to communication. Burnard and Morrison (1987) suggest that nurses are more comfortable with supportive, prescriptive and informative interventions than with those of confrontation, catharsis or catalysis. Yet, without exploration of a patient's real concerns, which may remain unexpressed for lack of 'permission' to speak, care cannot be effective or continuous. Interesting work has been done by Melia (1987) in investigating avoidance of communication which suggests that reluctance to confront patients' anxieties is related to issues of 'ownership' of information in a hierarchy. Communication is clearly a complex issue with repercussions well beyond the confines of learning specific skills.

However, for the purposes of giving patients 'permission' to express themselves, much can be achieved by the provision of time and privacy. Relatives need to be accorded the same consideration. Deliberately seeking knowledge of a patient's circumstances and feelings about returning home will let the patient know that this is a valued part of care and may dispel the reticence which can lead to gaps in provision. Staff are often diffident about approaching topics like finance, sexuality, spiritual need and death, and patients can be quick to pick this up and respond with silence. Sensitive questioning and following cues may elicit needs for information, counselling or referral.

## COMMUNICATION WITHIN THE PRIMARY HEALTH CARE TEAM AND WITH OTHER AGENCIES

Communication between members of a primary health care team is in as parlous a state in some instances as that between the primary and secondary sectors. The concept of the primary health care team developed and continues to be supported (Edwards, 1987) for the purposes of combining skills to produce a greater whole than the sum of those individual skills. In this way it is hoped to provide holistic and coordinated care. However, considerable communication difficulties are structured into the composition of these teams, related to the varying educational preparation, social status and gender of their members, and complicated by the different systems of employment within a team. Bond et al., (1987) found collaboration to exist but at a low level, with district nurse/general practitioner functioning closer than that between health visitors and general practitioners. Health visitors may feel the conflicts inherent in team working more acutely than district nurses because of the more autonomous nature of their practice and independent access to clients (McIntosh and Dingwall, 1978) and it is a common strategy in the management of teamwork problems to preserve apparent harmony by reducing communication (Hunt, 1979).

Communication within teams varies tremendously across practices. Hockey (1966) found that district nurses had access to too little information on patients and rarely paid joint visits with a GP, a practice that may still be continuing today. A major facilitating factor towards effective teamwork appears to be shared premises but although informal chance meetings between staff may increase interpersonal communication, interprofessional collaboration needs to be deliberately aimed for by all members of a team. Sharing recorded information, the identification of key workers to individuals or families, agreement on practice objectives and the analysis of role responsibilities are often areas meriting attention. Focused meetings on patient care, and the establishment of systems to inform all members of patients' movements in and out of hospital, may make an invaluable contribution to the continuity of care.

One area of concern is often the lack of contact with social services personnel. Otton (DHSS, 1974), emphasising the importance of personal links between health and social services staff, recommended that health centres should be designed to include accommodation for social workers. However, social worker attachment or alignment with primary health care teams is by no means the rule, and duplication of services and lack of coordination may be found. The recommendations of Griffiths (1988), that 'packages of care' should be developed and managed for individuals by 'care managers' and that community nurses may act as agents in this respect, has many implications for liaison between health and social services.

Paramedical support for the primary health care team is not well developed in many parts of the country. Patients must rely on the secondary sector for access to occupational therapists, physiotherapists, speech therapists, dietitians and so on, and members of the primary services may feel deprived of skills by lack of contact with these disciplines. Care is bound to be fragmented where one discipline works in virtual isolation from another. Many primary health care teams may also regret a lack of contact with representatives of housing and social security departments.

Communication between the primary health care team and the voluntary sector is often minimal. Many opportunities for gain from the direct services, self-help support or special expertise of client-group-related organisations are lost, and sources of revenue for patients may remain untapped through lack of contact with or knowledge of the fund-raising activities of local societies. The voluntary sector in turn has much to gain from communication with primary health care teams regarding the direction of funds to problems like incontinence which do not generally attract public attention or generosity. All primary health care teams need mechanisms, such as contact with voluntary bodies or community health councils, by which consumer opinion of services can be monitored.

## COLLABORATIVE SCHEMES

### Planned Early Discharge

Increasingly, early discharge following various types of minor and intermediate surgery has been the response of surgeons anxious to increase patient throughput and reduce waiting times for operation. Hockey and Buttimore's (1970) experimental study of such a scheme showed success in releasing hospital bed days without any apparent adverse effects on patient care or recovery, and indeed with some positive responses from patients especially regarding enhanced privacy. The care of postoperative patients is not, however, a large part of the district nurse's workload, and it is likely that the full potential of this area of her work has yet to be tapped. It has to be said that much early discharge is planned, if at all, in a rather reactive and piecemeal fashion, without due consultation with community services. Chisnell (1988) found that patients tended to be referred for specific care, but on assessment by the district nurse were often provided with extra care not requested by hospital staff, suggesting that planning and referral to services while in hospital may be inadequate.

District nurses are often keen to add to the variety of their caseload and to provide patients with the option for early discharge, but may be hampered by inadequate staffing levels, or by lack of confidence engendered by isolation from recent developments in hospital. With proper staffing establishments, technology to aid immediacy of response to patient need, and increased contact between hospital and district nurses, there is scope for a much greater involvement of the district nurse with patients undergoing, or preparing to undergo, surgery. Many patients on waiting lists have problems or disabilities, such as reduced mobility or obesity, to which the district nurse could make a contribution (Freeman et al., 1988). The assessment of social and environmental conditions relevant to recovery at home, advice on maximising fitness pre-operatively, information about forthcoming surgery, and planning with the patient for discharge are all interventions the district nurse is well placed to make to improve the continuity of care.

## 'Shadowing' and Exchange Schemes

An increased awareness of the potentials and problems of other nurses' roles is offered by schemes which seek to 'attach' individual members of staff from one area of patient care to those of another for a period. Student nurses are often subject to periods of observation along these lines, but there is much to be gained by extending the approach. District nurses receive patients from many different specialties with rapidly changing perspectives and technology, and need to maintain their education as well as to act as ambassadors for their part in the continuum of care. 'Shadowing' or exchange can lead to the development of professional links, exchange of ideas and appreciation of roles (Edgar and Bytheway, 1988). Wards and outpatient departments specialising in care of the elderly, oncology, neurology and general medicine and surgery are of obvious interest to the district nurse, but other areas of potential collaboration may be opened up by widening the scope. Hospital nurses, especially those newly recruited to a unit, should also spend time with community staff periodically, to afford insights into local services, priorities and problems, and to rekindle their awareness of their patients as people with lives beyond the hospital walls.

## Shared Care

Patients requiring long-term nursing sometimes have such care shared between hospital and district nurses. This may take the form of regular respite care in hospital, or an arrangement whereby a procedure such as a dressing is carried out for the most part at home but periodically in a ward or outpatient department. Communication may be very good where such an arrangement is planned with the patient, family, hospital and community carers, and often close informal relationships are formed to the benefit of all parties. The real needs of the individual and the particular skills and facilities of hospital and community must however be taken into account for this type of shared care to be fully satisfactory. It is sometimes the case that where planning and liaison are not well executed, care plans may be altered by hospital or district nurses without reference to each other, leaving the patient confused and with a sense of not being the centre of care decisions. 'Ownership' of a patient is a feeling that many nurses have trouble overcoming, and occasionally quite strong antipathies may develop. Hospital and district nurses need to make conscious efforts at the outset of such a partnership in caring to consider their own roles and how they are to knit together for the patient's benefit. Patients are sometimes found to be making costly, tiring and inconvenient journeys to hospital for care which may be more appropriately provided in their own homes or health centres. Too often, this is linked to a lack of confidence in the skills available in the community, which may be better dealt with there than by recalling patients repeatedly to the secondary sector. Where a leg ulcer clinic is in operation, for example, it may be profitable to involve or attach a district nurse who can provide input on her patients and in turn disseminate skills and knowledge acquired to the community.

Community hospitals, in which beds may be accessed by primary health care teams, and in which district nurses are based, seem to offer an environment in which the barrier between hospital and community is less impenetrable. Rigidity of staffing arrangements is often relaxed by the use of staff in both settings, and where a patient is admitted with nursing rather than medical needs there may often be more consideration accorded to planning for discharge with the patient.

## Liaison Roles and Specialism

With a view to improving continuity of care between hospital and community, a variety of liaison nursing posts has evolved with a plethora of differing responsibilities and authority.

One model type is the district nurse who is designated to visit wards on a regular basis to take referrals and provide input into discharge planning. Her brief may be based according to client group, for example the elderly, or to organisational concerns. The problem often encountered with this approach is that effectiveness is largely related to the timing and frequency of her visits. If she cannot, by virtue of her other commitments, be present at relevant medical ward rounds, for instance, her contribution to the decision-making process involved in discharge is bound to be limited, and she may find herself merely acting as a distributor of messages which would be better transmitted directly. A district nurse in this position is acting on behalf of her colleagues attached to other practices or neighbour-hoods, and may therefore find she has no personal knowledge of particular patients and can only represent community care in general terms.

Full-time liaison nurses may also find themselves undertaking clerical work (Edwards, 1987) which detracts from their potential as facilitators of continuity of care, and much depends on their autonomy and support from other disciplines. Increased awareness of the multiple problems of the elderly has led to the creation of geriatric liaison teams such as those described by Hall (1982) which by acting in an interdisciplinary way, and by visiting patients both inside hospital and at home, can achieve smoother and more individualised transfer.

The development of the specialist nurse has arisen, in part, in recognition of the problems in continuity of care faced by certain groups of patients. The value of continuing care by one person is often appreciated by patients who are cared for at home and in hospital by the nurse specialist in diabetes, stoma care, terminal care, continence and so on. However, there are drawbacks attached to a dependence on this approach. First, concentrating on specific patient groups may lead to a diversion of attention and resources from patients who do not fall into any rigid category. Second, there is concern that the job satisfaction and skills of the generalist workers in primary health care will be eroded by specialists taking over sections of their caseload. Support and liaison rather than substitution should be the basis of an approach by specialist nurses with the aim of devolving skills and care to district nurses by a thorough commitment to contact and education.

## Joint Health Authority/Social Services Schemes

Frequently, a patient's problems on discharge from hospital are due to an inextricable combination of physical, psychological, social and environmental factors, which are approached of necessity by more than one agency. Without liaison, there is room for duplication between health and social services, and sometimes role demarcation disputes occur to the detriment of patient care. Over-rigid policies about 'who does what for whom' can result in confusion for patients and staff, and waste of skilled time. District nurses, for example, may find it strange that they are prevented from teaching skills to social services carers which they would normally expect a patient's relative to perform. It is encouraging, therefore, that there are moves between health authorities and social services departments to rationalise their approach to the care of discharged patients and extend their joint endeavours to include an attempt at prevention of admission to hospital. The Darlington Community Care project (Stone, 1986) is an example of this type of scheme, in which 'hybrid' home care assistants give care to frail elderly people, having acquired training to meet the specific needs of each client identified by members of a multidisciplinary team. By accumulating information about the costs of care, evaluation and comparison between alternative services becomes possible. This may be the kind of initiative envisaged by Griffiths (1988) for the future management of community care.

## Voluntary Agency Schemes

The Macmillan nursing service is an example of the way in which voluntary organisations can work together with health authorities to promote continuity of care, and indeed other such client-group-related agencies often provide funding for the continuing education of specialist nurses. At a more direct level, organisations such as the Red Cross may be prevailed upon to fund and distribute items of equipment, and there have been attempts to harness voluntary workers for the provision of direct personal care with training by health authority staff. The larger bodies have the capacity to investigate need and care gaps on a national scale, but it may be the case that small local concerns need coordination and the right sort of integration with the statutory services in order for both sides to benefit fully. Voluntary agencies value their independence and contact with the grass roots, and have much to teach health and social services staff about consumer perceptions of services (Harrison 1978).

## THE WAY FORWARD

Clearly, while much of the quality of continuity of care rests with the individual practitioners at the clinical level, there are educational and organisational implications to be considered.

The process of socialisation by professional education produces many of the attitudes held by nursing staff, and has a bearing on their perceptions of their place in a continuum of care. The emphasis of future nurse education on normality, health and community-centred care should enable nurses to view their patients more holistically and to base their approach on a sensitive and realistic appraisal of individual and community strengths and limitations. A common foundation for all nurses may also discourage insularity and fragmentation of skills, and prevent the locking into career patterns which occurs today. It is to be hoped that in the future closer communication between professionals of different health disciplines may be engendered by the development of initiatives in joint learning. Placing nurse training in establishments of higher education should encourage a broader and more questioning approach to learning and may break down some of the cultural barriers which damage team working.

In the meantime, community experience for student nurses is often felt to be inadequate in its usual form. Brown (1986) describes a link scheme whereby students augment their community experience by following home an individual patient whom they have nursed in hospital. Developments such as this, extended to include trained staff exchange schemes, need to be more widely applied if continuity of care is to become a reality. A greater two-way flow of staff between hospital and community, and structured mechanisms for increasing personal contact between the two sectors should be facilitated by managers. Many nurses attending interest group meetings or post-basic courses discover that the opportunity to meet staff from other disciplines, grades or areas of nursing proves more fruitful than the content of the material presented. The will to communicate across the great divide is present; it is the 'permission' and expectation that this should occur which is sometimes lacking.

Identifying in-service training need and promoting educational and exchange opportunities need to be a large part of the role of the nurse involved in liaison. Developments in professional practice are also her concern. New forms of delivery of care are emerging, such as primary nursing. The accountability of one nurse for the total care of a patient has been claimed to produce closer nurse/patient relationships which in turn lead to improved clarification of problems (Wright, 1987). The liaison nurse is in a key position to detect implications for the continuity of care and to support initiatives as appropriate. She should be involved in setting standards: the analysis of structures and processes required to reach satisfactory outcomes should be seen across the whole spectrum of care and not isolated to hospital or community frames of reference. Helping staff to evaluate their own practice with regard to discharge planning and implementation may highlight deficiencies in service provision within the community. The liaison nurse, by working in an inter-disciplinary way, may be able to facilitate solutions. These may range from negotiating systems of transfer documentation to initiating mutual support groups, to researching the recovery experience, or to encouraging the inclusion of district nurses in pre-discharge case conferences. If a liaison nurse is to be effective in reducing the fragmentation of care, it will not be by acting as a carrier-pigeon, but rather by identifying critical elements of the discharge process and by drawing out the skills and motivation of the nurses already involved in patient care.

## References

Anderson J (1988) Coming to terms with mastectomy. *Nursing Times*, 27 January, **84**, 4, 41–4.

Armitage S K (1981) Negotiating the discharge of medical patients. *Journal of Advanced Nursing* **6**, 385–9.

Bliss M R (1981) Prescribing for the elderly. *British Medical Journal* **283**, 203–6.

Bond J and Bond S (1986) *Sociology and Health Care*. Edinburgh: Churchill Livingstone, pp. 211–13.

Bond J, Cartlidge A M, Gregson B A, Barton A G, Philips P R, Armitage P, Brown A and Reedy B (1987) Interprofessional collaboration in primary health care. *Journal of the Royal College of General Practitioners* **37**, 158–61.

Bonny S (1984) *Who Cares in Southwark?* London: Association of Carers.

Bowling A and Betts G (1984) Communication on discharge. *Nursing Times* **80**, 83, 44–6.

Brown F (1986) Putting the community in focus. *Nursing Times* **82**, 14, 44–5.

Burnard P and Morrison P (1987) Nurses' perceptions of their interpersonal skills. *Nursing Times* **83**, 42, 59.

Charlesworth A, Wilkin D and Durie A (1984) *Carers and Services: a comparison of men and women caring for dependent elderly people*. London: Equal Opportunities Commission.

Chisnell J (1988) District nurses' work with postoperative patients (Short Report). *Nursing Times* **84**, 3, 54.

DHSS (1974) *Social Work Support for the Health Service. Report of the working party* (Chairman G J Otton). London: HMSO.

DHSS (1980) *Inequalities in Health. Report of a research working group* (Chairman Sir Douglas Black). London: DHSS.

DHSS (1986) *Neighbourhood Nursing – a Focus for Care. Report of the community nursing review* (Chairman Julia Cumberlege). London: HMSO.

Edgar I and Bytheway A (1988) Information exchange. *Nursing Times* **84**, 13, 42–4.

Edwards N (1987) *Nursing in the Community: a team approach for Wales*, Review of community nursing in Wales (Chairman Noreen Edwards). Cardiff: Welsh Office.

Freeman T, Hawthorn P and Payman B (1988) The effects of waiting for major orthopaedic surgery (Short Report). *Nursing Times* **84**, 17, 61.

Griffiths R (1988) *Community Care: agenda for action*. London: HMSO.

Hall P (1982) Home – with care. *Nursing Times Community Outlook*, 9 June, 169–71.

Harding J (1987) Study of discharge communications from hospital doctors to an inner London general practice. *Journal of the Royal College of General Practitioners* **37**, 494–5.

Harrison B (1978) Camden old age pensioners. In V Carver and P Liddiard (eds) *An Ageing Population*. London: Open University Hodder & Stoughton.

Hockey L (1966) *Feeling the Pulse: a study of district nursing in six areas*. London: Queen's Institute of District Nursing.

Hockey L (1968) *Care in the Balance: a study of collaboration between hospital and community services*. London: Queen's Institute of District Nursing.

Hockey L and Buttimore A (1970) *Cooperation in Patient Care*. London: Queen's Institute of District Nursing.

Hudson B (1984) Who cares for the carers? *Health and Social Services Journal*, 5 July, 790–1.

Hunt M (1979) Possibilities and problems of interdisciplinary teamwork. In J Clark and J Henderson (eds) (1983) *Community Health*. Edinburgh: Churchill Livingstone.

Kratz C (1978) *Care of the Long-term Sick in the Community*. Edinburgh: Churchill Livingstone.

Lefever R (1981) Health services at home. In J E P Simpson and R Levitt (eds) *Going Home*. Edinburgh: Churchill Livingstone, pp. 281–92.

Luker K (1983) Goal attainment: one approach to evaluation. In J Clark and J Henderson (eds) *Community Health*. Edinburgh: Churchill Livingstone.

McIntosh J and Dingwall R (1978) Teamwork in theory and practice. In R Dingwall and J McIntosh (eds) *Readings in the Sociology of Nursing*. Edinburgh: Churchill Livingstone.

Melia K M (1987) *Learning and Working: the occupational socialisation of nurses*. London: Tavistock Press, pp. 80–101.

Neville R G (1987) Notifying general practitioners about deaths in hospital: an audit. *Journal of the Royal College of General Practitioners* 37, 496–7.

Osler W, see Stott (1983) *Primary Health Care*, op. cit.

Panel of Assessors for District Nurse Training (1978) *Curriculum in District Nursing for State Registered Nurses and Registered General Nurses*.

Parsons T (1951) see Bond and Bond (1986) *Sociology and Health Care*, op. cit.

Roberts I (1975) *Discharged from Hospital*. London: Royal College of Nursing.

Ryland R K (1981) The demise of dedication. *Journal of Advanced Nursing* 6, 6, 510–11.

Salvage J (1985) The Politics of Nursing. London. Heinemann Nursing.

Skeet M (1974) *Home from Hospital*, 4th edition. London: Macmillan.

Skeet M (1983) Continuity of care. In J Clark and J Henderson (eds) *Community Health*. Edinburgh: Churchill Livingstone.

Stein L (1967) The doctor–nurse game. In R Dingwall and J McIntosh (eds) (1978) *Readings in the Sociology of Nursing*. New York: Churchill Livingstone.

Stone M (1986) Home is where the help is. *Nursing Times* 82, 14, 31–2.

Stott N (1983) *Primary Health Care: bridging the gap between theory and practice*. Springer-Verlag.

United Kingdom Central Council for Nursing, Midwifery and Health Visiting (1984) *Code of Professional Conduct for the Nurse, Midwife and Health Visitor*, 2nd edition. London: UKCC.

United Kingdom Central Council for Nursing, Midwifery and Health Visiting (1986) *Project 2000*. London: UKCC.

Vaughan B and Taylor K (1988) Homeward bound. *Nursing Times* 84, 15, 28–31.

Victor C and Vetter N (1984) Use of community services by the elderly three and twelve months after discharge from hospital. *International Rehabilitation Medicine* 7, 56–9.

Wade B and Bowling A (1986) Appropriate use of drugs by elderly people. *Journal of Advanced Nursing* 11, 47–55.

Waters K R (1987a) Outcomes of discharge from hospital for elderly people. *Journal of Advanced Nursing* 12, 347–55.

Waters K R (1987b) Discharge planning: an exploratory study of the process of discharge planning on geriatric wards. *Journal of Advanced Nursing* 12, 71–83.

Williams K (1974) Ideologies of nursing: their meanings and

implications. In R Dingwall and
J McIntosh (eds) (1978) *Readings
in the Sociology of Nursing*. New
York: Churchill Livingstone,
pp. 38–44.

Williamson J, Stokoe I H, Gray S,
Fisher M, Smith A, McGhee A and
Stephenson E (1964) Old people at
home: their unreported needs. In
V Carver and P Liddiard (eds)
(1978) *An Ageing Population*.

London: Open University/Hodder
& Stoughton.

Wilson-Barnett J (1981) Reason for
selecting care. *Journal of Advanced
Nursing* **6**, 6, 508.

Wilson-Barnett J and Fordham M
(1982) *Recovery from Illness*.
Chichester: John Wiley.

Wright S (1987) Patient-centred
practice. *Nursing Times* **83**, 38,
24–7.

# 4.1
# The Realities of Liaison
## Jan M O'Leary

### EDITOR'S INTRODUCTION

Liaison nurses work in a number of ways. Many work in isolation and often on a part-time basis, performing their liaison function alongside their everyday caseload work. It is comparatively rare, therefore, to discover a liaison service like the one described here, carried out on a full-time basis by a team of three.

Liaison is seen to have a major coordinating function drawing together statutory and voluntary services and using multi-disciplinary meetings to ensure that information is accurate and up-to-date.

Linking information is seen as central to the role and function of the liaison team. Communication must be multi-directional, there-fore, and not confined to the more usual passage from hospital to community. For care to be continuous it is also important that those who have been caring for patients at home should be enabled to share their knowledge with hospital staff. Discharge planning, therefore, begins with information from the community on the day the patient is admitted to hospital, or earlier than that if possible.

In its essence, the scheme described in this chapter portrays liaison as an enabling service. Liaison should not be seen as detrac-ting from the responsibility that the individual nurse holds for her part in planning continuity of care. The liaison team does not take over the assessment of patients' need and discharge plans but augments the part played by hospital and community nurses them-selves, offering advice where necessary. Their central position to all services is crucial and their impartiality necessary to enable staff to appreciate and understand the perceptions of others with a dif-ferent viewpoint.

Ultimately, the aim of liaison is to improve communication between hospital and community services to the extent that their shared objectives will have the same intention and result in more effective continuing patient care.

## THE EARLY DAYS OF LIAISON

It is now more than 20 years since liaison nurses were first appointed throughout the country. The need for liaison was initially identified when hospitals commenced the 'early discharge schemes' by which patients were sent home within a few days of their undergoing surgery. They then required continuing care, for sutures to be removed and dressings changed. With the increasing numbers of all categories of patients transferring between hospital and home, it has become apparent that if the patient is to receive continuity of care, a well-defined link is required between nurses working in the hospital and those working in the community.

Where the employing authority has recognised the need for this link, it is equally important that the liaison role is clearly defined, so that the link has credibility. If the liaison nurses fill gaps which should be filled by other professionals the true worth of liaison will not be recognised and the erosion of other people's roles will create barriers. These will hinder the provision of a liaison service.

During the four years I was a district nurse I did not receive sufficient and timely information which would enable me to provide the continuing nursing care required by many patients on their arrival home. Therefore, these patients suffered unnecessary discomfort and sometimes additional stress. As a nurse I felt unprofessional in my approach and became very frustrated when I did not receive the information I needed. I welcomed the opportunity of becoming a liaison nurse and thought with my appointment the problems would be resolved and that continuing care would be ensured for all patients if it was appropriate.

On commencement in post my aims were to establish, on a district-wide basis, an effective communication link to ensure where it was needed continuity of care for all geriatric, paediatric and general acute patients on their transfer from hospital to home.

I wanted to promote a better understanding between hospital and community carers and to encourage a team approach towards the concept of continuity of care. I also hoped to encourage the careful multidisciplinary planning of discharges, particularly for patients requiring considerable continued care. It took four years to establish an effective communication link between voluntary and statutory personnel who provide care on a district wide basis. The link has now been forged by a team of community-trained nurses, who are based in the district general hospital. Systems have been implemented for collecting, collating and distributing information. Relationships have been established by recognising other people's roles and by helping them to understand the liaison role. Collection of detailed information relating to the transfer of patients is achieved on formal and informal bases. The majority of discharges, especially of the elderly, are now planned from the time of admission. Crisis intervention is decreasing and continuity of care is ensured.

## DEFINITION OF LIAISON

The definition of liaison is a bond or connection between two units. In nursing liaison it is an intercommunication link between hospital and community nurse carers.

Liaison is a frequently misunderstood concept, the main culprits being those liaison nurses who have failed to identify their own role.

They can see a need but do not know how to respond effectively and therefore give a specialised liaison service. This is when gaps are filled inappropriately and the nurses' own needs are met but the continuing needs of the patient are not identified. In some areas liaison nurses work individually or in isolation. I consider that the majority of people can work better if they relate to a peer group.

## THE LIAISON TEAM

Liaison team-work can be achieved by each member specialising in one area of work, but understanding the roles of the other members. This enables deputisation and provides the cohesion vital to the efficiency and continuity of a service which can then be given seven days a week.

To work in liaison it is necessary to have the vision that one day hospital and community staff will make a concentrated effort to work as a team. At the moment they often exist not just as two separate units but as two units pulling in different directions.

The liaison nurse identifies this from the position in the middle as a go-between. For the liaison service to be effective the liaison staff need to be objective in their outlook. They should have the ability to remain impartial. It is very important for them to listen to everyone's individual assessment of the patient's continuing needs and help the different disciplines to understand each other's viewpoint. It is important that no one view is promoted over the other. This means that the liaison nurse can act as the patient's advocate, if she can retain a balanced approach and resist pressure being exerted by misplaced loyalties. The liaison service should be jointly funded from hospital and community budgets and not separately by either.

The liaison nurse can help to narrow the gap between both professional and voluntary carers in the hospital and community if relationships are successfully established. Direct communication is without doubt the most effective but it is practically impossible to achieve and this is where the liaison communication link can be an efficient alternative.

## INFORMATION SYSTEMS

The passage of appropriate information is central to the liaison function. Systems and procedures for collecting, collating and distributing information need to be implemented. Once the 'mechanics' are installed, the links can become established and effective communication can take place. Referral forms for the exchange of written information are useful 'tools' and can become part of well-defined admission and discharge procedures. However, the passage of information is not sufficient in itself. It has to be collected systematically, In the scheme described here, a referral form is used and completed by the senior nurse on duty in the ward or department. For the majority of patients it is completed on the day of discharge, but it is completed earlier for those patients requiring a visit on the day the patient goes home. More advance warning is given for those patients requiring considerable nursing care.

The form is in triplicate on carbon paper. The top copy is placed in a sealed envelope and given to the patient to hand to the district nurse unless the information enclosed could cause the patient or relative distress or if there is a possibility of the form going astray. In that instance the top copy is handed to the liaison nurse for posting to the appropriate district nurse together with the second copy which the liaison nurse receives as a matter of course. The third is retained in the patient's notes.

The form is, of course, only as good as the person completing it. If it is started on admission it can be more easily completed. If the discharge is not planned the completion is likely to be hurried and important points may be missed.

The United Kingdom Central Council guidelines on drug administration (UKCC, 1986) clearly state that a nurse should not give any medicines/drugs without a dated and signed drug sheet to follow and check against the actual medicine supplied. Consequently, if a patient is not able to take or administer any drugs, the details must be included on the referral form and signed by the prescribing doctor prior to the patient's discharge. The community nurse will then receive it before administering the first medication or treatment. The patient is also given three days' supply of any dressings or lotions used to cover the transition period.

## COMMUNICATING IN LIAISON

The liaison nurse visits the wards and departments daily. This enables the contents of the referral letter to be checked and any additional information required to be collected. This is done before telephoning the district nurse for those patients requiring continued nursing care. Additionally, referral forms are completed for all patients over 70 years of age. The top copy is then sent to an appropriate health visitor by the liaison nurse to pursue as and when it is felt to be appropriate.

## PAEDIATRIC LIAISON

In the field of paediatrics there will be some referrals requiring active nursing treatment and these are made to the district nursing service using the same systems. However, as many of the admissions to a non-specialist paediatric unit are of a comparatively minor nature, most of the out-going information will routinely go to the health visiting section of community nursing.

Information supplied from community to hospital is just as important to maintain continuity of care and can also be conveyed on similar referral forms. It is only the community carer who can describe the nursing care that has been given in the home and the patient's capabilities within the home environment. Confidence can be gained from knowing that information which the carer alone can provide is contributing to the patient's care in the hospital. Community care information helps to identify problems early, particularly regarding those patients who have unsatisfactory social and environmental conditions. When all the patient's needs are clearly identified, a smooth transfer from one nurse to another is ensured, whether from hospital or the community. If detailed information is not given, the care provided cannot always be tailored to meet the patient's needs. A flexible approach is vital as the patient's needs will vary considerably. If good communication has taken place, however, the carer's awareness is increased, an accurate assessment can be made and the most appropriate continued care can be provided.

## METHODS OF COMMUNICATION

With the current available resources, communication is either by telephone or by post. These present systems enable a considerable volume of information to be passed between hospital and community nurses. Improvements can be made, however, with the use of advanced technology.

A facsimile apparatus can enable information to be exchanged speedily and accurately between all specialties. Relevant information can be distributed and it can provide the necessary cohesion vital for better patient care. Providing the transceiver is used only by professional personnel, confidentiality should remain as secure as the present postal and telephone systems. When patients are first discharged, their needs are greater and support more urgently required. Therefore, it is important to have an efficient communication link to ensure the appropriate carer receives as soon as possible the information relating to the patient's continued care.

## BARRIERS PREVENTING GOOD COMMUNICATION

Personal barriers can create the most intractable obstacles hindering the sharing of information. The 'mechanics' for sharing information can be efficient but the information will not be there to be conveyed if it is withheld. This occurs when relationships are not established between the different disciplines, or if there is a risk of offending, or if the information can be misinterpreted.

Liaison nurses can resolve some communication problems if they establish good relationships with both hospital and community personnel. An important part of the liaison role is to identify clearly other people's roles and help them to understand each other's in addition to the liaison role. The liaison nurse must be able to relate to individuals at the right level, so that they will feel safe and not threatened. Communication at a deeper level can then take place.

Relationships will not be firmly established and effective listening and empathy are prevented if personal issues and feelings are not overcome. Lack of self-awareness, poor manners and temper are sometimes displayed when staff are working under pressure. The liaison nurse should discourage rivalry between hospital and community nurses. It is also important that the liaison nurse never shows lack of interest or a negative attitude. It takes a lot of self-discipline, maturity and wisdom to retain the controlled impartial attitude which the liaison nurse must always present. This can however reap rewards when information is freely imparted and the liaison nurse is always kept fully informed by hospital and community colleagues.

## THE SHARING OF CARE BETWEEN HOSPITAL AND COMMUNITY NURSES

To begin to share patients' care there must be a real understanding of each other's roles; this in turn will result in a sharing of information relating to the patient.

Community nurses can help to promote an understanding of patients' needs in the context of their home, families and usual environment. They can help hospital nurses appreciate the social determinants of the patients' illnesses, and to make the patients feel more comfortable in the alien environment of the hospital. It is pertinent to the patients' care in the hospital that the community carers volunteer the information relating to the patients' capabilities at home. Problems can be identified earlier and this can avoid the delay in the recovery progress. Visiting the hospital provides the district nurse with the opportunity to read medical notes and the nursing care plan on the ward. This allows her own assessment of patients continuing needs to begin.

The liaison nurse can be someone with whom the community nurses can identify and can become a point of reference in the hospital. This does not mean that the community staff should be tempted not to visit the hospital. The liaison nurses should only represent them if circumstances prevent the direct carer from doing so.

Community staff who are infrequent visitors to the hospital soon begin to feel threatened by the hospital environment and this makes it more difficult for them to call in casually. When patients require considerable care it is very reassuring for them and their relatives to meet the district nurse who will be caring for them at home prior to discharge from hospital.

The peripatetic nature of the community nurse's work makes it difficult for her to communicate directly with the ward staff on a daily basis. The liaison nurses should, therefore, be based in the hospital. With their community background knowledge they are able to intercede on the community carers' behalf. They are also able to obtain information from the direct care worker. If sufficient information is given when the patient is admitted it means that the community nurse can initiate the discharge planning. The information can be passed on a similar referral form to that used by hospital nurses when the patient goes home. The ward staff can then commence their assessment of the patient's continuing needs based on the additional knowledge of the care which the patient has received prior to admission. Again, the liaison nurse can ensure that the information is passed to the appropriate nurse.

## DISCHARGE PLANNING

Hasty, unplanned discharges are only defensible if genuine aftercare is assured. It is of great importance that sufficient, accurate information is collected, collated and conveyed to the appropriate community carer, prior to the patient's discharge. A weekly multidisciplinary

ward meeting provides an ideal situation for the exchange of information. These meetings are attended regularly by a member of the
medical and nursing staff, social work department, occupational
therapy, physiotherapy and liaison staff. The planning of discharges
and the subsequent communication require active input from all
members of the hospital multidisciplinary team. The timely involvement of the formal and informal home carers is equally important.
Whenever possible, patients' views should be represented. We must
not take away the responsibility they have for themselves. In certain
circumstances a trial home visit with the occupational therapist, prior
to discharge, also enables an assessment to be made by the appropriate community carers. These home visits are usually made with
patients who require considerable continued care, additional equipment and/or structural alterations, which will enable them to retain
optimum independence. When a patient requires considerable continued care which is to be provided by several different agencies it is
very helpful if the key worker is identified. This is the person who provides most care, for example the community nurse. The key worker
can then be a point of contact for all disciplines involved. This avoids
duplication of tasks and is less confusing for patients and relatives.

Where statutory community services are unable to meet the
increasing demands, voluntary agencies are now providing some of
the essential care which can include bathing, dressing and transferring the patient from bed to chair. Today they are included in the discharge planning, and have become the key workers in many cases.
There have been several patients who have been able to go home
when 'Relative Relief' and/or 'Crossroads' have offered their services. If these agencies had not been able to provide a substantial
back-up service, some patients would have remained in hospital.
When I initially came into liaison, voluntary agencies only provided
carers who were the 'icing on the cake'. Today they are often an
essential ingredient.

## THE LIAISON NURSE'S CONTRIBUTION

The liaison nurse can contribute to the continuity of care by acting
as a coordinator between the different disciplines and by keeping
everyone well informed. In liaison work, good personal relationships
with all members of staff make the two-way exchange of information
easier. This improves the standard of continued care for patients of
all ages. Visits to the liaison department should be included in the
orientation programme for all newly appointed trained nurses so that
the discharge procedure can be explained. It is equally important that
the liaison nurse is invited by the nurse education department to talk

to learners. The opportunity is then provided to give the nurses enough insight to think about continuity of care; the transfer of the patient rather than the discharge. The word 'discharge' seems very final and makes the concept of continuity of care difficult to grasp. Within a credible liaison service, transfer planning will be monitored and liaison nurses will ensure that all members of nursing staff really do consider continuity of care.

Needs are greater and support more urgently required (especially for the elderly) during the period when patients are first discharged. Unplanned discharges, therefore, are unacceptable and the liaison nurses encourage careful planning to enable appropriate community care to be provided. In the protective environment of the hospital ward elderly patients often imagine they will be able to manage at home and the expectations of their own capabilities may be unrealistic.

If the discharge is planned, appropriate aftercare can be identified which is suitable to meet the needs of the individual. The appropriate carers can then be included in the discharge planning.

The level of coordination required to make a discharge work is necessarily high if several carers are involved with assisting the same patient. The coordinator can be the liaison nurse. It should be pointed out, of course, that the sheer number of discharges of elderly people precludes community-based staff from attending all planning stages for every patient. This is where the liaison nurses can represent their views and give advice on which suitable community services are available.

## OBSTACLES HINDERING DISCHARGE PLANNING

Patients who insist on self-discharge can confound the discharge plan, but we should remember that everyone has the 'right to fail'; the elderly can have misconceptions about their ability to cope. When a patient insists on going home against medical and nursing advice, we should ensure that continued care is provided in order to avoid unnecessary risk. Within a relatively short time the patient may accept that he has not recovered sufficiently to be at home and may then agree to be readmitted, having come to terms with the loss of independence.

Relatives, friends and neighbours who encourage early discharge by confirming that they will fill the 'caring gap' should make us wary since, in reality, they often represent an unreliable resource, however laudable their voiced intention. This sometimes happens when the patient has a determined and strong personality. The people filling the caring gap may have been persuaded that the patient is more self-caring than is really the case. There are also cases where 'emotional blackmail' is used and the carers are made to feel guilty about the patient's hospitalisation. Where considerable care has been provided prior to admission by relatives, neighbours and friends, they should be included in the discharge planning and invited into the case conference. They can then identify the assistance which is being given to the patient in hospital and listen to the multidisciplinary assessment of the continuing care that will be required.

The shortage or lack of sufficient community services and aids available can also delay discharges. More resources are obviously necessary, especially in the face of growing numbers of very old and vulnerable people. It is highly desirable that the majority of elderly patients will continue to be discharged back into their own homes. Their independence should be encouraged and maintained for as long as possible. Not all elderly people will need aftercare support, but many will need some assistance if only in the short term.

As with the elderly, general/acute wards have their own special problems. Many patients admitted for planned surgery are discharged rapidly following operation and ward staff have a tendency to gather less information at the admission stage than they might do. Planning for discharge may therefore take place against a background of minimal data.

It must be said that a rapid turnover of patients does not provide sufficient time for nursing staff to gather all the details which complete the whole picture in order to assess adequately the continuing needs of the individual. On acute medical wards, home visits are frequently requested to be made on the same day as the patient is discharged. Newly diagnosed diabetic patients receiving twice daily insulin therapy are fairly common, and even when the patient is administering the medication it is desirable that professional support is provided when the injection is given at home for the first time.

The level of communication from the liaison department needs to be high so that community nurses have sufficient notification when an evening visit needs to be undertaken.

Accident and emergency, day care and out patient departments and fracture clinics can present problems too. Patients attend these areas for short periods only and a lack of understanding of the role of liaison in relation to the problems encountered in the departments may lead to little or no thought being given about what might occur when discharge has taken place: a patient living alone, for example, with an arm in plaster or dislocated shoulder may find it difficult to undress.

Forward planning for continuity of care, therefore, remains just as important in all areas.

# TO IMPROVE THE CONTINUITY OF CARE

## Patient Involvement

Good communication with the patient is equally important. Written instructions should be given to all elderly patients, before they leave hospital, giving details of their medication, guidance for self-care and also the services which are to be provided for them after discharge together with a list of useful telephone numbers and addresses for a wide range of community-based services. The patient needs to be counselled about taking medication correctly. Considerable success has been recorded where patients have been given the opportunity to administer their own medication on the ward as part of their rehabilitation programme.

In my opinion, when elderly patients who do not require continued nursing care are discharged home, a mandatory visit should be made by a member of the primary health care team within the first 48 hours of discharge, especially to those patients over 75 years and living alone. Following a period of hospitalisation, loneliness can be felt more acutely. A further visit should then be made by a member of the primary health care team about one month after discharge to check on long-term recuperation. A reassessment of the service provided and evaluation of care given would be especially useful prior to any outpatient follow-up appointment. It would be a major step forward if liaison nurses could always ensure that there is a timely response to provide the care needed for all patients when they transfer between one environment and another.

If the words *discharge* and *admission* of patients were replaced by *transition* of patients perhaps there could be 'Always Continuity – Never Crisis Intervention', and nurses in the hospital and community would identify themselves as a nursing team with the same objective, and not as two separate services pulling in different directions.

## Bibliography

DHSS (1986) *Neighbourhood Nursing – A Focus for Care*. Report of the Community Review (Cumberlege Report). London: HMSO.

HAS/DHHSI (1986) *Report of Care of the Elderly in West Suffolk*. London: HMSO.

O'Leary J and Thacker P (1985). Blueprint for liaison. *Nursing Times*

*Community Outlook*, May, 40–3.

O'Leary J (1988) A period of transition. *Nursing Standard* **2**, 43, 51.

Potterton D (1984) The yawning gap (Hospital to Home 3). *Nursing Times* **80**, 32, 34–5.

UKCC (1986) Administration of Medicines. A UKCC Advisory Paper. London: UKCC.

# 4.2
# Paediatric Liaison and Health Visiting
## Bridie Fuentes

### EDITOR'S INTRODUCTION

In this chapter, Bridie Fuentes describes her work as a paediatric liaison health visitor in South Gwent, an urban area in the south-east of Wales. She describes how the liaison scheme began in the 1970s and its development since its inception. The need to create an efficient service was important for the part-time liaison nurses, who also carried a health visiting caseload. A number of ways of making the channels of communication more efficient are described.

Much time was spent establishing and building good relationships with other staff members, since productive relationships with medical, nursing and ancillary staff are crucial to effective communication. The involvement of the child and its family at various points in the series of communications is emphasised.

As other writers have noted, the problems caused by patients being discharged home on Friday are great. Information is not passed from hospital to community staff easily at the end of the week, and patients and their families are often left without the support they crucially need at this time.

Finally, the implications for the development of the role of the paediatric liaison health visitor are considered in the light of their acknowledged contribution by families and professional staff and questions posed about the appropriate means of funding the post which bridges caring in both hospital and at home.

## THE ROLE OF THE PAEDIATRIC LIAISON HEALTH VISITOR

The role of the paediatric liaison health visitor (PLHV) is one of creating a two-way channel of information so that staff can provide more effectively good patient care. The service must be there to benefit the patient and not the community or hospital staff.

The work of the PLHV can best be explained by showing how one district general hospital and its community are served.

The Royal Gwent Hospital is a district general hospital in Newport and serves a paediatric population of 54,500 in South Gwent (total population is 320,700). The service began in the early 1970s when it was realised that children were being admitted and discharged from hospital without the family health visitor's knowledge. Copies of hospital discharge letters to general practitioners (GPs) were received but usually too late to be of practical use in supporting families. It was decided, therefore, that designated health visitors should attend one clinic a week and also visit the paediatric wards to see the patients' records. Joining the consultants' ward rounds was tried but proved wasteful of health visiting hours in terms of what was gained.

Following NHS reorganisation in 1974, it was realised that the paediatric liaison service had considerable potential for expansion, but because of budget restrictions development was limited.

Each PLHV covered the sector of the county in which she was based and attended the special care baby follow-up clinic as well as having a caseload of up to 300 families with children under school age. In the course of ward visits to copy information from patients' records, it became apparent that talking to ward staff was of greater value. At the same time, recognising the overlap in health visiting and social work, the hospital social work department requested regular weekly meetings between ward staff of the special care baby unit (SCBU), paediatric unit, hospital social workers and health visitors. By then the PLHVs were working up to three sessions a week in liaison.

In addition, an important and helpful new component of the service came into being. Ward clerks in the two paediatric wards telephoned clerks in each community sector on Monday mornings and informed them of any child admitted over the weekend. Each morning the child's name, date of birth, address, GP and provisional diagnosis were given by the community clerk immediately by telephone to the family health visitor who could then inform the ward staff of anything that might be relevant to that child's care while in hospital. The hospital clerk also made a list of the children admitted through the week for the PLHVs. (This was later discontinued as unnecessary.) More recently, because of heightened awareness of child abuse in the wake of cases of non-accidental injury ending in tragedy (DHSS 1974 and 1975) the accident and emergency department (A & E) has become another contact for the PLHV. A form has now been produced which gives details of all children under the age of five who attend the department, including GP referrals. These forms are distributed to the family health visitor on a weekly basis, and she then decides whether a follow-up visit is necessary. The forms are kept in the child's visiting record and any new health visitor will be able to see at a glance the number of hospital contacts that child has had and the reason for the visits, i.e. whether for frequent accidents or because the A & E department is being used as a GP's surgery. Parents may need educating in home safety or help with problems to which they are trying to draw attention like poor health, housing or personal relationships. In one case a single mother with three children under two years attended the A & E department every time one of the children had a fall in an attempt to call attention to her need for rehousing. Sometimes the nursing staff in the A & E department may feel some concern about a child. Such concerns may refer to the parent's attitude, or to the unusually high number of times a child has attended. A senior nurse then contacts the PLHV to express her concerns in order that the family health visitor can visit and give more support if needed.

Currently, in the light of increased pressure on hospital beds, together with greater accent on community care and the cost-efficient use of staff, the paediatric liaison service is being reappraised. Certain groups of children are targeted for increased support in the community. These include children with diabetes mellitus, cystic fibrosis, tracheostomy or requiring nasogastric feeding. This has meant further clinical teaching and study days for the health visitors involved.

To summarise the present service:

1. Each of the three sectors in Gwent, Islwyn, Torfaen and Newport, has 1–3 PLHVs who meet hospital nursing and social work staff weekly to exchange information about children in hospital. At the weekly meeting, admissions and discharges from SCBU are also discussed and the information passed to the family health visitor, as it is she who will be giving on-going support to the family. The PLHVs carry a caseload and spend up to three sessions a week on paediatric liaison.
2. Each of the three consultants has a health visitor attending special care, diabetic/metabolic, cystic fibrosis and assessment clinics. The names of those children who persistently fail to keep their appointments are given to the family health visitor and followed up.
3. The names of all children admitted to hospital are passed to the family health visitor by clerks on a daily basis.
4. The PLHV collects weekly from the A&E department the forms relating to all children under the age of five who have attended there.

5. Special attention is given to any child with a long-term or chronic condition and his/her family before and after discharge from hospital.
6. Health visiting colleagues use the PLHV to obtain information and answers to their queries from the paediatric consultant about the children they visit. The consultant also uses the PLHV to gain information from the family health visitor about families whose children are seen in the paediatric clinic.
7. The PLHV frequently finds it necessary to explain to parents what a consultant meant during the clinic consultation, for example, interpreting medical terms. She may also find herself providing tea, sympathy and information when parents have just been given bad news.

## DISCHARGE FROM HOSPITAL AND THE ROLE OF THE PLHV

### Assessment of Patients due for Discharge to Community Care

In the case of the diabetic child, the PLHV is informed of the child's admission and diagnosis as soon as possible and will arrange to see the child with the parents before discharge in order to introduce herself, discuss any worries, and assess how much support will be necessary and who will give it. Further discussion then takes place with the ward sister and dietitian and the likely date of discharge obtained. The PLHV at this point contacts the family health visitor to discuss which of them will give daily support until the family gains confidence in diabetic management. As a general rule, the child who is under school age is best supported by the family health visitor who can use the PLHV as an information source if necessary. The PLHV may invite her colleague to a diabetic clinic as a way of updating and informing her of the individual consultant's management policies. The family health visitor may also visit the ward and talk to the family, child and ward staff if she is to undertake the support in the community.

When discharged the child will take home a checklist of the teaching programme so that it can be seen at a glance what information the child and parents have been given. There is a different checklist for diabetes, nasogastric feeding, tracheostomy and intravenous antibiotic therapy for the children with cystic fibrosis. If the liaison or family health visitor's knowledge about any procedure is deficient, she is invited to the ward and taken through the procedure before the child goes home.

## Subsequent Involvement

The family is usually visited or contacted daily by telephone for as long as necessary and any problems discussed. Parents quickly gain confidence and expertise and do not become dependent on the health visitor to give support.

If the child attends school, both the teaching staff and the school nurse are informed and any possible difficulties discussed before the child returns to school, for example, how to deal with hypoglycaemia as this frequently causes great anxiety in teachers.

Diet will also be mentioned, but the dietitian will contact the school directly to explain the child's needs with the staff.

Having provided home support, the PLHV is in a position to report to the consultant any problems that may be developing and if possible prevent them from becoming worse. Alternatively, a clinic appointment may need to be brought forward because a mother, health visitor or GP is concerned.

Many patients are seen regularly in clinic and a relationship is built up with parents who will sometimes confide in the PLHV some of their worries which they may consider too trivial to tell the consultant. These can usually be resolved during the consultation.

## Difficulties that May be Encountered

Successful liaison is dependent on good communication and teamwork. If any member of the team, from consultant to clerk, is not committed to making it succeed for any reason then enormous difficulties are created. For example, it has occasionally been found that consultants are reluctant to release clinical details of a patient to health visitors on the grounds that it is a breach of confidentiality. A compromise can usually be found, though the service will be less efficient. This is more likely to apply to consultants who are not paediatricians and unfamiliar with the work of health visitors.

Health visitors doing liaison work need to remember that they are visitors to a ward and should always present themselves to the nurse in charge, saying why they are there and being prepared to be flexible if the ward is very busy.

Planned discharges, where community staff have been informed and suitable arrangements made for a patient's care in the community, are often impossible if a ward has been filled with emergency admissions and parents are pressing for their child to go home. It is not unknown for a child being fed by nasogastric tube to be discharged on a Friday afternoon without prior warning. The nursing officer then has the impossible task of trying to contact a health visitor to provide support, on a day when the health visitors are only at their bases for the first part of the morning.

Yet another problem is that of incorrect information being passed to community staff. The address on hospital records may not always be the current one. In one instance a twelve-year-old girl was sent home for a weekend and the district nurses were informed by the PLHV as she needed considerable nursing care. The child's address had changed. An irate district nurse was unable to locate the patient and the mother was unable to manage unsupported. The child had to be readmitted to hospital.

Even worse is a failure to inform community staff of the death of a child in whose care they may have been involved. No system is entirely foolproof but any nurse who has been caring for a child who has died should think about who may be involved with the family. Only then can the situation be avoided in which appointments are sent to bereaved parents, or a health visitor arrives at the child's home to do a developmental test. This breakdown in communication is more likely to occur when a child has been transferred to an intensive care unit or to another hospital for specialised treatment.

## RELATIONSHIP WITH OTHER COMMUNITY AND HOSPITAL STAFF

### Consultants

The PLHV who attends clinics has a valuable learning opportunity. She will gain knowledge of the individual paediatrician's ways of managing diseases. This information can then be passed on to community staff. Over a period, mutual trust and respect are built up and the health visitor's area of expertise is recognised and valued.

### Nurses

Hospital and community nurses are working on the same side; namely, the patients'. The role of the PLHV is not always fully understood. Hospital nursing staff should feel able to discuss with the PLHV all aspects of community care prior to a child's discharge, but PLHVs are still occasionally confused with social workers, possibly because they are seen at meetings with the social workers and do not wear nurses' uniform.

Nursing staff on the paediatric wards of the Royal Gwent Hospital recognised the need for more community paediatric support nursing some years ago, and in 1986 they made a good case for employing a hospital-based paediatric support nurse who would visit patients at home and carry out nursing procedures normally done in hospital. The aims were to reduce the length of hospital stay and the number of readmissions as well as giving support to parents at home. Community nurses and health visitors were, however, unhappy about this as they felt they had community training and experience and were well able to support families nursing children at home, providing good planning was done before a child was sent home.

## Medical Records Clerks and Medical Secretaries

Close cooperation between the PLHV and medical records staff enables hospital records to be updated when patients move, change GPs or change their names. Appointments can be brought forward, for example, if parents are anxious about their child and feel that it is too long to wait until the next appointment, or cancelled. The family health visitor can inform the PLHV, who will then ask the hospital clerk to make the appropriate change. Reports from community staff will be filed in a patient's records if given to the clerks. Cooperation benefits both PLHV and the clerical staff.

## Social Workers

A close working relationship can develop with hospital paediatric social workers because of the overlap in their roles in the area of working with families with problems and the fact that they also visit families at home.

## Dietitian

The dietitian gives the PLHV valuable help and advice on a number of conditions, for example, diabetes, phenylketonuria or coeliac disease. The PLHV will frequently introduce the dietitian to her health visiting colleagues so that she can give them advice about monitoring and management of diets.

## Nursing Officers

The role of the PLHV is sometimes in conflict with her other duties and the nursing officer for health visiting will occasionally feel she has to curb her enthusiasm in order to maintain a balance between the two roles. This brings into question the whole subject of liaison work and whether there is a need for a nursing officer for liaison itself.

However, the PLHV can often provide helpful information quickly on children in hospital as well as definitions and guidelines on the management of various diseases. The nursing officer spends more time at her office base and can be a more accessible community contact for the hospital staff. The relationship therefore is partly one of mutual support and partly one of conflict.

## Health Visiting Colleagues

The PLHV's colleagues use her as an information resource and as a line of enquiry. Health visitors and community doctors will often use the PLHV to ascertain from the consultant a child's suitability for full vaccination. For example, it may be necessary to ask whether to omit pertussis from the immunisation course when there have been problems in the neonatal period or to ask about the need for physiotherapy where there are motor problems. Colleagues may report on difficulties that families are experiencing and these can sometimes be resolved without the need for a clinic appointment. Feeding problems are frequently discussed as it is important that all who are dealing with a family are giving the same advice.

## Mental Handicap Team

Information about mentally handicapped children in hospital is passed to the health visitor of the mental handicap team so that support can be given to the family by someone known to them. Details of a child newly diagnosed with mental handicap are usually passed to the team on a more formal basis by the consultant.

## District Nurses

The district nursing sister is less frequently in contact with the PLHV because parents are usually taught any necessary procedures that need to be carried out in the home before the child leaves hospital.

## SPECIAL PROBLEMS

A number of problems demand attention and are beginning to be recognised by both community and hospital staff. Not enough has been done due partly to the separation and fragmentation of hospital and community services and partly to financial constraints.

## Need for Better Support of the Adolescent Diabetic

The newly diagnosed diabetic is offered some community support by either the PLHV or the family health visitor. Paediatricians would like to see much more support given, not only to the newly diagnosed diabetic child but also to the adolescent diabetic who often has many difficulties. Not all parents have insight into the upheaval of adolescence. There is not always time in the clinic to talk at any length and many teenagers attend on their own. If a diabetic liaison nurse or health visitor experienced in diabetic care were able to visit and counsel the family in their own home and send a report to the consultant, his knowledge of that family would be much more complete, enabling better care for the child also. Greater cooperation between hospital and community will also help the patient become independent sooner. The teenager who fails to keep appointments may be denying the condition. It is possible to have poor control of diabetes and still feel fairly well. As a result he may stop testing his blood glucose levels and fail to appreciate the long-term need for regular monitoring which helps to maintain good health and prevents admission to hospital in a crisis, as so often happens. With home visiting and closer support this risk would be reduced.

The family with a diabetic teenager has virtually no support outside the hospital at a time when they probably need it most. The transition from child to adult is rarely smooth even without having diabetes. Some health authorities have recognised this and arrangements are made to see the young people at a time or place which they find more acceptable.

## Need for Respite Care for the Mentally Handicapped

At present severely mentally handicapped children are admitted periodically to paediatric wards to give their carers a much needed break. Now that greater emphasis is being placed on community care (Secretary of State for Wales, 1983) little seems available for this area of need. Admitting these children to an acute ward is inappropriate as it exposes them to infection unnecessarily and places more demands on a hospital's tight budget.

## Need for Unsocial Hours Cover

Children are most frequently discharged from hospital at weekends when health visitors and their nursing officers are off duty. This will mean that either the hospital is contacted if problems arise and the child is readmitted or a nurse from the district nursing service unknown to the family is asked to call. Someone is needed like the PLHV, who is known to both hospital and family and who could visit and give advice and support.

## Communication

When a death occurs in hospital there can be a delay of as much as a week before the family health visitor is informed. Hospital staff do not always appreciate that bereavement counselling by the family health visitor is long-term and is more effective if it can begin soon after the death has occurred. Radio-paging devices could be a useful way of locating the PLHV in such cases.

## SOME POSSIBLE SOLUTIONS

Some of the recommendations in the Report of the Review of Community Nursing in Wales (Edwards, 1987) are particularly relevant to paediatric liaison work:

1. Nursing services are needed outside normal working hours (8.6).
2. Liaison staff should provide an educational service to colleagues in both hospital and community (8.28).
3. Respite care should be provided on both a day-to-day basis to relieve carers for a short period and periodically for a day or weeks at a time (8.33).

Problems of caring for a child at home do not only occur between 9 a.m. and 5 p.m. and parents have to contact the hospital unless their family health visitor has, unofficially, given them her home number.

Liaison staff are already providing a limited educational service to their community and hospital colleagues. It could be expanded in a formal programme of continuing education for all nurses.

Paediatric liaison work has been allowed to evolve naturally in an informal way. It is fitted in often with quite large caseloads. These need to be reduced to a more realistic level. Individuals in the field have been left to develop the service as they feel appropriate within loosely defined limits. Although this freedom has some advantages there comes a time when the service can develop no further without management support. Separate management of liaison staff would facilitate further development and provide the necessary support.

Health visitors and hospital nurses need to be more aware of each other's jobs: joint study days are an obvious solution. These might include such specific subjects as the management of particular diseases and more broadly, discussion on a team approach to continuity of care.

The paediatric liaison role needs to be considered alongside that of the liaison nurse for the elderly or mental handicap liaison health visitor: they work as members of a team and are managed separately from general family health visitors.

We need to question whether the time has come for shared funding of the paediatric liaison service with the hospital and a more formalised job description. At present hospital staff are uncertain about how far the role of the PLHV extends. To have the job clearly defined would help staff to use her more effectively for the ultimate benefit of the patient.

The work that the PLHV does is recognised by paediatricians, hospital nursing staff and community as being worth-while and they are all asking for an extension of the service. It seems that we are only scratching the surface of this area of need.

If funding could be increased and even shared by hospital and community then a paediatric liaison team could be set up, consisting of a number of community-based health visitors working half their time in liaison. They would retain a small caseload and so maintain their knowledge of the local community. Unless this area of need is recognised and given more importance, the service provided by PLHVs cannot develop. This can only be detrimental to good continuity of care.

# References

DHSS (1974) Report of the Committee of Enquiry into the Care and Supervision provided in relation to Maria Colwell.

DHSS (1975) Report of the Committee of Enquiry into Provision and Co-ordination of Services to the Family of John George Auckland.

Secretary of State for Wales, Nicholas Edwards (1983) *All Wales Strategy for the Development of Services for Mentally Handicapped People.* Cardiff: Welsh Office.

Edwards N (1987) *Nursing in the Community: A Team Approach for Wales* (Chairman Noreen Edwards). Cardiff: Welsh Office.

# 5
# Beyond the Barriers: Towards Integration

Roger Deeks

## EDITOR'S INTRODUCTION

The distinction Roger Deeks draws between a community hospital which is primary care team-led and a neighbourhood hospital which is regarded as an offshoot of a district general hospital and consultant-led is an important starting point in the discussion of an integrated service. The barriers to integrated care are acknowledged and the examples given of the crossover of nursing in the community and in community hospitals serve to remind us of important ways in which integration of care can be achieved. Conversely, they point up the problems that prevent this being achieved in alternative settings. Implicit in this approach is the relinquishment of the 'ownership' of patients in any particular setting. It is replaced with a need to acknowledge the supremacy of the patient and the primacy of the patient's home over institutional care. The care the patient receives is paramount; where the care is received is secondary. In response, the carer gives the care in whatever setting is most appropriate for the patient. This is an ideal to which many nurses would aspire. Many will argue that it is not possible to achieve, perhaps because of the type of care required or the location of hospital care. The principles, though, need to be considered against a future of shorter hospital stays, increased community care and an ageing population.

Flexibility and integration are essential for continuous care in whatever setting the patients happen to be placed.

## ORGANISATION FOR CARE

This chapter is concerned with the organisation and management of nursing services within community or neighbourhood hospitals and the communities which they serve. The physical scale and ease of access characteristic of the smaller hospital permit face-to-face interaction between hospital and community nurses. These features also facilitate the smooth transition of patient care between hospital and home. This can be contrasted with large hospitals where there is frequently a break in care and communication, due in part to their size and function and relationship to the community.

The management of care and care providers in a small-scale setting, involving both community and hospital scenarios, can be more intimate, personal and unobstructed by any type of bureaucratic overlay. From both the clinicians' and managers' perspectives there is the opportunity for imaginative and innovative development of nursing practices.

Any discussions should begin by recognising that there are many different types of small hospital. Unlike district general hospitals which evolved to fairly consistent patterns, most smaller hospitals are survivors of cost-cutting exercises and short-term planning expediencies. Historically, little attention has been paid to the role and function of small hospitals. Indeed the number and distribution of small hospitals has only recently been identified by the Association of General Practitioner Hospitals (Cavanagh and Jones, 1985). Since the publication of a DHSS circular (1974), the precarious position of small hospitals in Wales has substantially changed. Community hospitals are now recognised as an essential component of service provision. This has led to an investment in small hospital building programmes and the development of many existing hospitals. Some small hospitals have become extensions of primary care, transcending the normal arbitrary division between primary and secondary care, and contrast with others that are seen as peripheral units associated with a district general hospital, to which patients requiring long-term care are referred.

The characteristics of what are sometimes called 'neighbourhood' hospitals are substantially different from 'community' hospitals by virtue of their relationship to the district general hospital and the community (see Figure 5.1). Community hospitals tend to have their main input from the primary health team, who are responsible for admitting, managing and discharging their own patients. Neighbourhood hospitals tend to be off-shoots of the district general hospital, taking transfers prior to discharge, and are hospital consultant-led.

The DHSS circular (1974) described the aim of a community hospital as being:

> to provide appropriate medical and nursing care to those patients who cannot be reasonably cared for in their own homes (patients are not expected to require highly specialised treatments, or investigations), . . . to provide acute, respite, long-term and terminal care for patients as near as possible to their own homes so that they can be visited more easily by friends and relatives, and so that relatives can participate in the patients' care, as appropriate.

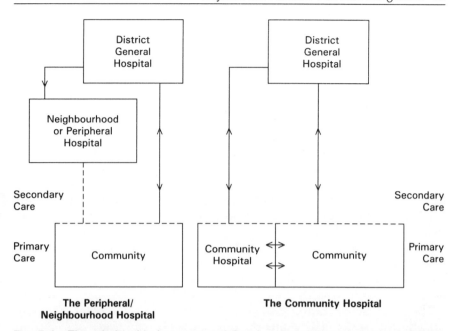

The Peripheral/
Neighbourhood Hospital

The Community Hospital

**Fig. 5.1 The relationship between peripheral, community and district hospitals and the community.**

From the previous discussions and these prescribed aims of a community hospital, it is reasonable to suggest that its functional role and, most importantly, its size and relationship to the community, allow it to bridge the interface between hospital and community care. The scale of the hospital, and the intimacy of working relationships between staff in and outside the hospital, minimise the 'care gap'. This is, of course, dependent on how care and services are organised. It should be acknowledged that many of the principles and practices of integrated services can be provided by large hospitals, and the claim that integrated care is only possible in small hospital situations is not tenable. However, it can be stated that the scale and purpose of community hospitals make integration more practicable and achievable.

A useful starting point for any discussion of integrated care is the recognition (see chapter 1) of the fact that nursing care is provided in hospital and at home by two very different groups of nurses. Although simplistic, this statement in itself acknowledges the first major difficulty in providing integrated care.

A community nurse's professional development only begins after completion of a career as a hospital nurse. Consequently, nurses become qualified community nurses only when they have succeeded as hospital practitioners. Some nurses enter the community area because the conditions of service suit their social commitments. Despite the background and varying degrees of commitment to the concept of community care, community nurses quickly acquire a homogeneous identity. Change, therefore, particularly the planning of 'integrated services' which might involve an alteration in the number of hours and patterns of working, can be threatening to the identity of staff groups and their established conditions of service.

The integration of services can be undertaken in a number of ways. There is the potential for rotating staff, employing 'integrated' staff who can work in either hospital or community, operating a primary nurse system where one nurse is accountable for a patient's total care (Manthey, 1980), or using hospital facilities as work bases for community staff.

Rotation of staff can be undertaken at any level. However, with qualified staff the need to meet statutory training requirements must be recognised. This may require a major training investment on behalf of management.

The practice of rotating staff should never be employed in a manner that dilutes skills. The main purpose of such a strategy is to create a unified team approach. This need not necessarily involve use of a primary nurse concept, merely periodic role change. Given time, it is possible to build up an approach and framework common to both settings. There is no doubt that the community nurse learns to set objectives on a partnership basis with patients and families. The home and the hospital are markedly different health care settings with quite different role relationships: 'Naturalistically, the family is "captain of the team", by mere virtue of having choice in who is allowed to enter their private domain' (Chapman and Chapman, 1975: 74).

In a community hospital there is often a strong commitment to respite care and symptom relief in terminal care, all of which should be done in partnership with patients, carers and their families. The goal, therefore, is to make the hospital the patient's home. It is precisely the nurse–patient relationship that exists in the community that is required in the hospital setting. This will enhance hospital care and the transition to subsequent community care. Staff with a community training and experience fully appreciate the need to teach carers and patients how to care and cope for themselves. Staff without this experience find it difficult to share the care in a hospital setting.

Wilce (1986), in describing the work of the Lambeth Community Care Centre, states the underlying philosophy with regard to patient–nurse relationships thus:

What the centre's staff most want it to be is a secure base from which people who care or have been ill, can manage their own recovery, adaptation and living – or sometimes, dying. This way they can go home knowledgeable and confident rather than helpless.

The difficulties of the hospital nurse adapting to this shared care role relationship, which is more developed in the community, are compounded by patients' expectations. The 'sick role' is a well-defined sociological concept, which has been discussed by Parsons (1951) and others. Patients' expectations of hospital often equate with dependence and being 'told what to do'. Pre-admission counselling, information booklets and thorough explanations on admission can all help to prepare the patient and family. The patients must never be given the impression that they are being left to go it alone. They must be assured that they are entering a contract, a partnership, to assist them through illness, recovery or dying.

Chapman and Chapman make the following observation of an advocacy model of helping: 'the behaviours of the health care advocate are primarily dependent on the patient and the situation in which both encounter one another. Reinforcement of helpless, voiceless, dependency behaviours of patients can be avoided as assets, or strengths, of patients are acknowledged and utilised in growth-enhancing ways from the outset' (Chapman and Chapman, 1975: 60).

The other important partner in this contractual relationship is the carer. In the context of community care, the Welsh Community Nursing Review, 'Nursing in the Community – a team approach' (Edwards, 1987), acknowledged the role of carers. The need is stressed for professional care providers 'to work in partnership with the people they help, and not to see themselves as benevolent superiors'. The need for partnership, as outlined in this report, is an essential lynchpin of good community care.

Wilce (1986) observed that staff at Lambeth had to realise that 'they are doing a better job, not a worse one, if they leave most of the practical caring to a husband who has moved in [to the hospital], with his dying wife, with unobtrusive skilled help only now and then.'

If we achieve the right balance of relationships between nurses, patients and carers, the environment, be it hospital or home, becomes the only variable and a backdrop to the activity. To achieve this philosophy of care, much of the hospital culture which is counterproductive to an individualised approach must be overcome.

It becomes relevant, particularly in view of Wilce's observation from Lambeth, to ask how the decision is reached on where the patient should be cared for. Discharge and admission become an informed agreement between the nurse, patient and carers. In many situations involving the chronically sick, disabled and dying patient, the three principal parties will be the patient, carer and nurse. In others, where there is a significant treatment component, there may be a medical input.

In community hospitals the management of bed use and decisions on admission and discharge are primarily a nursing prerogative. The use of 'rotation beds', that is, respite or relief care beds, should above all be a nurse/patient/carer decision. Policies on use of respite beds should be agreed jointly between the hospital/community staff and carers' support groups. A carers' group is an invaluable form of self-help and regulator/arbitrator for use of scarce resources.

To summarise the discussion so far, it can be argued that the nature of admissions and discharges, because of the type of hospitalisation, is substantially different in a community hospital from those to and from district general hospitals. The relationships between nurses, patients and family/carers is the same in the hospital as in the community, particularly if staff are brought together and where possible interchangeable.

The following case example provides one illustration of admission and discharge 'policy' in a community hospital:

Mrs Jones, aged 39, had advanced carcinoma of the uterus. The medical objective of treatment had altered from a curative one to that of symptom relief. Mrs Jones had a supportive husband and three children, aged 10, 16 and 17. The patient was committed to maintaining her role in the home for as long as possible. Her district nurse introduced Mrs Jones to the community hospital and sister-in-charge as a pre-admission exercise. She was first admitted with the objective of pain control and providing rest and nourishment. She was nursed in a sideroom suite, and visiting and participation in her care was agreed with her family.

Following her first admission, it was agreed that any future admissions would be arranged at short notice on request of the patient or her district nurse. Mrs Jones' care plan, admissions and discharges were all mutually agreed. She was admitted three more times. Her periods of admission were all relatively brief, the main purpose being to use the hospital services to relieve her symptoms and re-establish her at home as quickly as possible. On one occasion she was admitted immediately, at her own request, because of nausea.

Her district nurse participated in her hospital care and her plan of care was a mutually agreed document by all parties. The general practitioner was also closely involved and committed to the plan of care.

Mrs Jones' care plan followed her in and out of hospital during this time. Mrs Jones died in hospital with her family present and the team continued to support her family for sometime thereafter.

This brief sketch illustrates how continuity and quality of care involving both home and hospital care can be maintained throughout a period of need.

A further barrier to integrated care is when there is a disparity between hospital and community formulated nursing goals and objectives. Hospital staff will frequently ascribe problems and prioritise them without due deference to the patients' beliefs and wishes and their home environment. This dimension of care planning was discussed by Goodman:

> In hospital, nursing tends to be orientated to the acute situation that has necessitated a patient's admission. The aim of care is likely to be cure, and success can be defined in terms of the patient's recovery and subsequent discharge. The focus of hospital based nursing is, therefore, towards short-term care planning – with discrete, clearly defined goals. (Goodman, 1987).

Goodman is concerned that hospital-trained nurses will apply the same values in the patient's home, thereby having a particular difficulty in dealing with dying or chronically sick patients and long-term physical, social and emotional support. However, it is reasonable to assume that the danger that Goodman perceives, that is, the transfer of values, can work in the opposite direction. The community trained and experienced nurse can take into the hospital setting a whole new set of values, perspectives and frameworks from which to approach patient care. This is particularly true of the community hospital, where medical input is from GPs who frequently share a more holistic view of the patient and adopt a less autocratic position regarding nurse–patient and family-directed care planning. GPs working in community hospitals have a responsibility to the patient, both in and out of the hospital, unlike their hospital counterparts, who can afford to take a very narrow, medically-oriented view of the individual, with responsibility being limited to their in-patient care.

The principles of staff integration and blurring of boundaries can produce common standpoints on models of nursing, goals and objectives, transcending both hospital and community nurse groups and care settings. In this situation, debate about discharge documentation becomes irrelevant. Care plan documents become a common resource applicable and viable in both settings.

It is useful to consider some of the practical implications of integrated care. The primary nurse concept can be used to promote integrated care. This has been particularly successful with services such as those for the elderly mentally ill which are provided in some community hospitals. The greatest problem is separating management of care from the provision of care. So long as the primary nurse directs care and remains accountable for it, the actual provision can be delegated to other staff if required. Community nurses can, in the right circumstances, manage the care of their patients throughout their stay in hospital. Frequently, it is of enormous benefit to the patient if community staff participate in the provision of that care for a period after admission and prior to discharge. Joint staff meetings between hospital and community nurses, carers and volunteers on admission is a good practice preparing patients, carers, relatives and staff for meeting problems through the span of required hospitalisation and later at home. In respite care situations it is advisable to bring community staff into the hospital to care for the patients they would otherwise be seeing at home. This maintains continuity on every level and is also a good use of resources. Carers have reported a major improvement in the quality of services they receive and feel much less guilt when allowing their relatives to be admitted. They feel confident that the standard and level of care that is provided at home will be maintained.

It is possible for some staff to provide care in both settings. Day hospitals are a particularly important focus for use of staff who work in both the community and hospital in the same day. Staff visit their own patients prior to the day hospital opening to assist patients with washing and dressing and assessment of other activities of daily living. This gives the day hospital team an invaluable insight into planning appropriate courses of action for patients when they are fully conversant with the home environment. In a small-scale setting, this can be an economical use of limited resources.

In concluding this chapter it must be acknowledged that the divisions between hospital and community care are seen only as arbitrary lines that mark changes in the setting for health care. Differences become minimal if some of the nurse–patient relationships based on our respect for persons is transferred from the community into hospitals. Organising groups of staff to share each other's experience will help achieve short-term goals of integrated care. However, the future depends on re-orienting nurse education to produce a practitioner equally competent in the home and the hospital.

## References

Cavanagh A J M and Jones R H (eds) (1985) *Association of General Practitioner Hospitals Handbook and Directory*. Brecon: Malcolm Jones Association for AGPH.

Chapman J E and Chapman H H (1975) *Behaviour and Health Care*. St Louis: C V Mosby.

Department of Health and Social Security (1974) *NHS Development of*

*Health Services: Community Hospitals*. London: DHSS (Circular HSC(IS)75).

Edwards N (1987) *Nursing in the Community – a Team Approach for Wales*. Review of community nursing in Wales (Chairman Noreen Edwards). Cardiff: Welsh Office.

Goodman C (1987) Nursing care of the chronically sick in the community. In *Handbook of Community Nursing*. Newbourne Group.

Manthey M (1980) *The Practice of Primary Nursing*. Boston: Basil Blackwell.

Parsons T (1951) *The Social System*. London: Routledge & Kegan Paul.

Wilce G (1986) The better approach. *The Guardian*, 14 May.

# 6
# The Liaison Complex

Sarah Jowett and Sue Armitage

## EDITOR'S INTRODUCTION

'Liaison' is a word that has slipped into general use in nursing and is common currency when considering the link between hospital and community. It implies adequate links between people. Considered under the umbrella of communication, it no longer appears simple and clear-cut. The efficacy of liaison lies in the quality and type of information given and the facilitation of its further use. Liaison is not unidimensional. The personal attributes of the individuals liaising and their interpretation of it affect how it is developed and played out.

Liaison thus can be seen as a 'link-up' between two areas, and the individuals within them as a channel for the communication of information. It is multifaceted and can best be described as a complex having a number of features which are offset against how it is played out.

Communication, which is central to effective discharge planning, does not occur in isolation from how nurses in hospital and nurses in the community perceive each other and how they feel about the others' work. In other words, it concerns their awareness and understanding of the others' role and function in that part of the organisation within which they work.

The responsibility for the quality of continuing care need not rest with any one individual. Liaison is a concept that can be regarded differently by nurses in varying situations.

The research study described in this chapter set out to examine what liaison meant in the continuity of care. Three groups of nurses were interviewed throughout the Principality of Wales: liaison nurses; senior nurses with joint management responsibility for both hospital and community nurses in the rural areas; and a sample of hospital and community nurses.

The transfer of patient care between hospital and community nurses and the function of liaison enabling that does not rest solely on the variety of transfer documents that may or may not be used. Fundamental to how nurses interact with one another and their patients are the beliefs they hold. The intention was to examine the underlying perceptions which ultimately affect how care is given.

Increasing numbers of liaison nurses have been introduced, and the debate that is taking place on how they should function is reflected in the findings of the study reported.

The majority of nurses would agree that direct nurse-to-nurse communication is the ideal to work towards. But many nurses would also argue that in practice it is not possible for hospital nurses to contact a district nurse or health visitor about each patient to be discharged and that a liaison nurse is necessary to effect better continuing care for patients.

A choice has to be made. If it is decided to appoint liaison staff then a number of implications ensue. The research findings reported below relate to certain areas crucial to the development of an effective liaison role.

## BACKGROUND TO THE STUDY

There has been a marked increase in the introduction of liaison nurses in the United Kingdom as a move to improve continuity of care. Despite the many suggestions for developing these posts (Amos, 1973; Continuing Care Project, 1975, 1979, 1980), there has been no systematic assessment of their contribution to continuity of care. Subjective reports describing the role of the liaison nurse have been published (Reid and Waddicor, 1970; Gordon, 1983), but apart from small-scale studies by Paxton (1974a and b), Warner (1981) and Tuplin (1984), no systematic evaluation has taken place.

It was this situation that prompted a two-year research study, begun in September 1985, to explore the area of hospital–community liaison and the role of the liaison nurse in Wales. The study highlighted a Liaison Complex illustrating the many and varied aspects of liaison. This chapter focuses on the results of the study and, in view of these, makes suggestions about ways of improving the continuity of care (Armitage and Jowett, 1988).

Before focusing on what the Liaison Complex involves, the research design of the study is described.

### Research Design

In a complete evaluation programme the elements of structure, process and outcome are usually explored (Donabedian, 1969, 1980, 1982; Weiss, 1972). In this study of hospital–community liaison, the focus was on the process and structure of liaison schemes, with attention to outcomes given in a second stage of the research.

As initial enquiries indicated that process and structure features of liaison schemes were diverse and almost unpredictable, it seemed appropriate to adopt a grounded theory approach (Glaser and Strauss, 1967). Rather than beginning research with preconceived ideas, this approach aims to collect information about what is happening in the 'real' world and to develop a theoretical explanation of it. Data were collected by focused interview (Merton and Kendall, 1946). Key aspects of the process and structure of liaison were identified from the literature and incorporated in an interview guide. This guide was not regarded as inclusive but as an *aide-mémoire* in exploring respondents' experiences of liaison.

The sample included 196 respondents. This incorporated all designated generalist, paediatric and geriatric liaison nurses in Wales (n = 45), together with all senior nurses having a liaison remit within their joint hospital–community management posts (n = 27). Equally representing the nine health authorities in Wales, a random sample of hospital sisters (n = 62), district nurses (n = 31) and health visitors (n = 31) were also included.

Within the grounded theory framework, data analysis involved studying the taped and transcribed interviews to identify key trends, themes and categories of material. Elaboration of these categories enabled a theoretical explanation of the data to be developed and highlighted the Liaison Complex which is the focus of this chapter.

## The Liaison Complex

The Liaison Complex represents the liaison process with the factors affecting it (Jowett and Armitage, 1988). The structure of liaison affects the process and is therefore seen as integral to it. Structure, then, is included as one of the many factors affecting the liaison process. The key elements of communication and discharge planning comprising the liaison process are affected by the three major concepts of community awareness, attitude and organisational factors. The elements and the concepts which have an effect on them are interlinked in what may be described as a complex of liaison (see Figure 6.1).

### Elements of Liaison

1. Communication between nurses working in the hospital and community settings.
2. Discharge planning: the planning of a patient's discharge and immediate aftercare, before the date of leaving hospital.

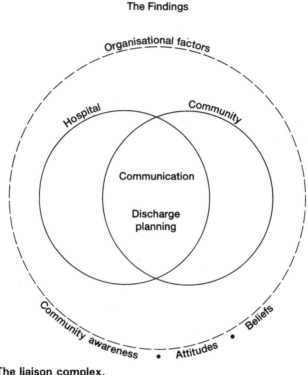

**Fig. 6.1   The liaison complex.**

*Concepts Affecting Liaison*

1. Community awareness of hospital staff. This includes knowledge of community services, perceptions of the roles of community-based professionals and recognition of the effects of home background on patient care.
2. Attitudes of hospital staff to the concept of continuity of care and its importance in patient care.
3. Organisational features of patient care, which affect the liaison process.

The Liaison Complex was manifested in different ways according to the setting in which liaison was taking place. The nurses in the study described liaison as occurring in three different ways. From these descriptions, three models of liaison were identified.

*Model 1*

In this model, liaison occurred directly between nurses working in community hospitals and those working in the community. No liaison nurses worked in this setting but senior nurses had hospital management responsibilities, with an incorporated liaison remit. This model was predominant in rural areas, where community hospitals are common. These hospitals care for patients requiring non-acute medical and nursing care. They are locally-based with patients requiring acute care travelling to more specialised district general hospitals. In most community hospitals, medical care is given by general practitioners and admissions and discharges frequently managed by nurses.

*Model 2*

In this model, liaison occurred directly between nurses working in district general hospitals and the community setting. No liaison nurse was involved.

*Model 3*

Liaison occurred indirectly between nurses working in district general hospitals and the community setting. Liaison nurses were involved in patient transfer.

## COMMUNICATION AND DISCHARGE PLANNING IN DIFFERENT SETTINGS

Within the Liaison Complex, communication and discharge planning are the two key elements in the process of liaison. In this section, the two elements are examined and the way in which they occur in different settings is described.

### Communication

*On Admission*

Communication around the admission period was more frequent in community hospitals (Model 1) than in any other setting. Communication in this setting was normally on an informal basis and was usually face-to-face or occasionally by telephone. Hospital nurses were satisfied with the quality of information received.

In contrast, information was rarely transferred when patients were admitted to district general hospitals (Models 2 and 3). In these settings, communication was described as 'patchy' or 'hit and miss', though it was more likely to occur if the admission was planned.

Information transfer initiated by community nurses was difficult because they were rarely informed of unplanned admissions.

The liaison nurses in the study were involved in transferring information between hospital and community nurses. None had much routine involvement otherwise, and the emphasis was on information transfer on discharge. Respondents saw this as satisfactory because the most problematic period for patients was seen to be the discharge period.

## On Discharge

On discharge from community hospitals (Model 1), communication was satisfactory. In spite of their liaison remit, senior nurses rarely had any involvement and communication was normally directly between hospital and community nurses. Referral information was considered to be appropriate, comprehensive and well-timed in relation to discharge. When patients were admitted to hospital, communication was normally verbal, either on a face-to-face basis or by telephone.

However, communication on discharge from district general hospitals (Model 2) was regarded as unsatisfactory. Thirty-five (56 per cent) community nurses (20 health visitors and 15 district nurses) felt that the information they had was often inappropriate and lacking in quality and quantity. Some nurses also complained that certain patients requiring community care were never referred for it. District nurses complained that they received little warning of discharges which seemed to be due to lack of forewarning in planning discharge dates. One senior nurse commenting on discharges from district general hospitals said: 'If [the patients] need a hoist, bed cradle or commode, it takes a while because our stores come from a central point. At least, if they gave us a few days' notice . . .'

The methods of communication used within Model 2 also posed problems. Written communication was used most frequently and, apart from the occasions where nursing process documentation was transferred, was seen as the least effective. Respondents suggested that the transfer of nursing process documentation should be encouraged, although attention is needed to practical issues. Problems about the loss of records and their ownership were raised. Telephoned and face-to-face communication was regarded as most effective but was rarely used.

In Model 3, all liaison nurses (n = 45) had a role in transferring information on discharge. Twenty-one liaison nurses (46 per cent) compiled lists or transferred scant biographical information about patient discharges. Although this was felt to be useful, it was not considered to require the skills of a trained nurse. This was particularly well illustrated by one liaison nurse:

'I just sit there and write down the name, age, diagnosis and GP of every child. It means wading through notes and copying facts down. I think the other staff find it useful otherwise they would never hear about someone who was taken in and who had gone home. But it is a clerical task really. I don't think it needs a health visitor to do it.'

Most of the liaison nurses in the sample had some role in passing more substantial information between hospital and community staff. Although these referrals were viewed as both comprehensive and appropriate, respondents felt their effectiveness was hampered by a time-lag and that a degree of information distortion often occurred. Information distortion was well illustrated by this comment from a district nurse:

'I get referrals from liaison nurses which are great on things like if meals-on-wheels are ordered and if a commode is needed. But it is difficult for them to include things about expressions and moods and things. You can't get that sort of thing over in writing very well.'

Time-lag was described by community nurses (a health visitor and district nurse, respectively):

'You see the problem is that the liaison officer only goes into the ward on Tuesday afternoons. Then say a child is sent home on Wednesday, we don't hear about it for 10 days. Sometimes, the sister will ring us if it is something urgent, but I'm sure some get missed.'

'Half the time, I go round the liaison nurses and ring the ward myself. You have to otherwise messages just never get through in time.'

Liaison nurse involvement in transferring referral information was likened to the game of Chinese whispers by some respondents:

'There are these party games that you can play where you say the same word and pass it all round a group of people and by the time the information gets to the end of the group, it is nothing like the information that was fed in at the start and I think this can happen very much in liaison work. This is why I see my role as triggering things off. I much prefer to encourage the health visitor responsible for the family to contact the ward sister directly.'

Referrals from liaison nurses were also seen as removing responsibility from hospital nurses which led to complacency about their involvement in information transfer.

One way of reducing some of the problems identified was when liaison nurses acted as facilitators in direct nurse-to-nurse contact. These liaison nurses acted as advisers to nurses on information transfer and discharge planning. This was considered effective because a third party was not involved between hospital and community staff. Consequently, information distortion and time-lag were less of a problem and hospital staff retained the responsibility for initiating communication on discharge.

### Discharge Planning

Community-based respondents were generally satisfied with the discharge planning that took place in community hospitals. Senior nurses, although having a liaison remit, rarely had direct involvement (Model 1). Discharge planning began early during the period of hospitalisation and the quality was satisfactory.

Although respondents recognised that slower patient turnover allowed more time for discharge planning to take place, the widespread involvement of community nurses, the positive effects of community awareness and attitudes towards discharge planning were all felt to make an important contribution. In contrast, community nurses, liaison nurses and senior nurses felt that although discharge planning in district general hospitals (Model 2) had improved in recent years, problems still existed. Echoing past studies (Skeet, 1970: Gay and Pitkeathley, 1978; Armitage, 1981), respondents felt discharges continued to be poorly planned both in their timing and the follow-up arrangements made. A senior nurse familiar with discharges from district general hospitals stated: 'Patients come home on Friday evening needing walking aids, frames and bedpans. On Friday at 3.30 pm or 4 o'clock, it is impossible to get anything.'

In Model 3, all liaison nurses (n = 45) had some involvement in discharge planning, although the pattern of their involvement was variable. Community nurses felt problems experienced with discharge planning were less prevalent if a liaison nurse was involved, but that improvement was possible. Some respondents felt that liaison nurses were taking over discharge planning, and that collaborative planning between nurses involved in direct care would be more appropriate. Respondents felt liaison nurses should develop an advisory role to overcome this. They considered that hospital nurses should be encouraged to plan discharges effectively themselves and that community nurses should be more involved when appropriate.

## FACTORS AFFECTING LIAISON

### Concepts Affecting Liaison

As described earlier, liaison is affected by three major concepts:

1. community awareness of hospital nurses,
2. attitudes of hospital nurses,
3. organisational factors of patient care.

In liaison between nurses in community hospitals and the community (Model 1), successful communication and discharge planning reflected the positive attitudes and community awareness of hospital nurses and at the same time displayed some contributory organisational features.

In contrast, liaison between nurses in district general hospitals and the community (Model 2) reflected negative attitudes, poor awareness of community care and some organisational problems. Where liaison nurses were involved in liaison (Model 3), it is clear they have positively affected these otherwise negative factors.

It was found that the physical and ideological closeness of the hospital and community sectors of care are the key factors affecting community awareness, attitude and the organisation of liaison.

To enable better understanding and to focus upon the way forward, a discussion of the physical and ideological closeness of care is required.

### Physical Closeness of Hospital and Community Nurses

Liaison between nurses in community hospitals and the community (Model 1) was characterised by a unique physical closeness, minimising organisational barriers between them and positively affecting community awareness and attitudes towards continuity of care. Physical closeness was particularly well illustrated in this interview with a district nurse (DN).

> DN 'We get on so well with them at the local hospital [community hospital], we are like a team, I suppose. . . . We know what they want and they know what we want . . . there is no "them and us" between us.'
> I 'Has it always been like this?'
> DN 'Ever since I've been there. It wasn't like this when I worked near [district general hospital]. We never knew any of the staff there. I suppose we could have gone in, but we didn't. We were very suspicious of them. I suppose we trust each other here.'

In this setting, physical closeness is attained by three common features:

1. hospital and community nurses are based in the same building,
2. integrated hospital–community posts,
3. hospital–community staff exchange programmes.

These features rarely existed in Models 2 and 3, where liaison was between nurses based in different buildings and often separated by geographical distance. Liaison in Models 2 and 3 was also characterised by separate hospital and community clinical posts and consequently the lack of cross-fertilisation of ideas and experiences. In contrast, physical closeness in Model 1 allowed nurses to communicate effectively on a face-to-face basis.

In Models 2 and 3, the physical segregation of hospital and community nurses meant they could rarely communicate informally. Consequently, they relied upon written methods or the telephone, which were seen as less effective.

Hospital nurses had limited contact with community colleagues. To effect liaison they relied largely on nurse training which had been oriented towards hospital and was therefore limited in knowledge of community matters. Changes in basic nurse education were stressed as a fundamental requirement in order to improve continuity of care.

Because liaison nurses were trained community nurses, they were able to influence their hospital colleagues' attitudes and awareness of community. Where they used their experience to advise and facilitate in direct hospital community nurse liaison, their role was perceived positively.

However, in contrast, where liaison nurses took over responsibility from their hospital colleagues for communication and discharge planning, they had what could be described as a superficial positive effect, but which did not extend to a deeper level. They had a useful 'bridging' function in providing an effective link in communication and discharge planning, but taking on this responsibility meant that hospital nurses became less proficient and motivated in initiating liaison themselves.

## Ideological Closeness of Hospital and Community Nurses

In liaison between community hospitals and the community (Model 1), nurses in both settings were jointly managed by one senior nurse. This signified a unified approach to care and stimulated a positive attitude towards liaison. In contrast, within Model 2, hospital and community nursing services were separate and signified a segregated approach to care. Consequently, hospital nurses developed an ambivalent attitude towards continuity of care.

Where a liaison nurse was involved (Model 3), the post was symbolised as a move towards unified care. The role was frequently described as a 'link' or 'bridge' between the hospital and community sectors and helped to foster awareness of continuing care.

**Structure of the Liaison Role**

The liaison nurse makes an important contribution to the continuity of patient care and it is appropriate therefore to discuss some of the structural aspects of the role, which, according to those nurses involved in the study, are most influential in its effective functioning.

*Part time/Full-time*

Most liaison nurses had a part-time commitment to the role but felt that a full-time commitment would be more effective.

*Availability*

Respondents felt that ease in contacting liaison nurses was most important in their effective functioning. Availability was variable but the following factors were felt to increase it:

● a recognised office base,
● regular work pattern of liaison nurse,
● easy availability by telephone,
● availability by a bleep or answer-phone system.

Combining the role with a community post:
   Many part-time liaison nurses combined their post with a district nursing or health visiting post. Many of them experience difficulties in combining the two posts and suggested this practice should be discontinued.

*Establishing the Role*

A firm establishment of the liaison role within the organisation was viewed as important in its effective functioning. Respondents identified a number of key issues affecting this and made suggestions about how it could be improved. These will be discussed in the last section of the chapter.

*Getting to Know the Job*

Many liaison nurses perceived problems in 'learning the ropes' of the post and felt it was a major issue in striving for effective functioning. Most of the problems related to introductory guidance given to post holders and the frequent lack of peer support.

*Base and Employment of Liaison Nurses*

Liaison nurses were based in both hospitals and the community. The most important factor related to this seemed to be their availability to others. Although many varied suggestions were made about the future location of liaison nurses, both hospital and community-based respondents felt that a hospital base would be most effective.

All the liaison nurses in the sample were employed by the community nursing services. Respondents felt this to be the most appropriate employing authority because they felt hospital employment would symbolise accountability to the 'hospital organisation' and could result in losing 'community orientation', which is perceived as fundamental to the role.

*Professional Background of Liaison Nurses*

All the liaison nurses in the sample were qualified community nurses; some were from a health visiting background, some from district nursing and some from both.

In posts attached to paediatric units, respondents felt that a health visiting or district nursing qualification combined with specific paediatric experience was essential for liaison. However, for all other liaison posts, community orientation was felt to be the most important feature and therefore either district nursing experience, health visiting or preferably both were perceived as important.

*'Attachment' of the Liaison Nurse*

The patterns of liaison nurse attachment varied. A common problem was that groups of individual patients were being missed by liaison nurses. To rectify this, respondents felt that, depending on the size, attachment to a complete district general hospital or a manageable sector of one would be most practical.

*Meeting the Needs of the Organisation*

The degree of flexibility granted to holders of liaison posts was variable. Respondents felt that flexibility within the role is crucial to its effectiveness, especially if the role is to move from the referral-nurse to facilitator-nurse pattern of practice. The respondents believed that liaison nurses should be allowed flexibility within the role to enable adaptation to the dynamic needs of the local organisation and population.

## FUTURE OF LIAISON

Three models of liaison have been identified. They can be viewed along a continuum reflecting the extent of effective continuity of nursing care for patients leaving hospital to return home. The three models range from the best continuity in Model 1 (community hospital to community) to Model 3's variable effectiveness with the contribution of a liaison nurse to the least continuity in Model 2 (district general hospital to community with no liaison nurse).

In considering the future we have two polarised choices. Either we develop liaison between hospital and community with direct collaborative discharge planning or we opt for the intermediary role of an individual nurse liaising between the two settings. Whichever option is chosen needs developing.

The study identified three areas of change which could lead to more effective continuity of care:

1. educational changes to improve community awareness and attitudes towards continuity of care,
2. organisational changes,
3. changes in the liaison role.

### Educational Changes

Among hospital nurses based in district general hospitals, poor awareness of community and attitudes towards it affected their ability and motivation to effect continuity of care.

### Basic Nurse Education

Respondents felt that although emphasis on community care within current educational programmes is more satisfactory than in the past, potential for improvement remains. Typical comments from senior nurses were:

'It isn't so much the lack of teaching, it is the emphasis. If they [students] spent the initial part of their training outside the hospital, they would realise that home is normal and hospital is abnormal.'

'Well, I feel that the whole training is predominantly based in the hospital, when really, more care goes on in the home. Patients only go into hospital for brief acute periods, don't they? Students need to realise that patients spend more time at home.'

The following changes were suggested:

- Clinical and theoretical aspects of community care should be introduced at the beginning of educational programmes.
- The specific study of community care should be extended in duration. One liaison nurse commented: 'The students have three-month blocks of surgery and medicine etc., so why not three-month blocks in the community? There just isn't enough importance attached to it.'
- The concept of continuity of care and aspects of community care should be stressed as a *core* element throughout all basic nurse education.

### Post-basic Education

In addition to changes in basic nurse education, respondents suggested changes in continuing education are needed to encourage more effective continuity of care. For hospital nurses the development of post-basic courses in community care could contribute towards improved liaison.

### Educators and Managers

In addition to curriculum changes, respondents felt continuity of care would only be fully effected if educators and managers developed more community awareness and positive attitudes towards community care. Respondents suggested that nurse teachers and nurses in hospital management posts should be encouraged to develop a greater awareness of community nursing.

## Organisational Changes

Where not already operating, direct communication between hospital and community nurses would greatly improve continuity of care. The following changes would enable the two groups of nurses to liaise more effectively:

- moves towards hospital and community nurses being based in the same building,
- the introduction of integrated hospital–community clinical posts,
- the development of hospital–community staff exchange programmes,
- the provision of up-to-date directories of local nursing services and other facilities on all wards (this could be the responsibility of liaison nurses),

- the introduction of locally agreed improvements in written and telephone communication channels (as suggested by Edwards (1987), attention should be given to the use of computers, car radios, telephones and 'bleeps' for community nurses).

### Role of Liaison Nurses

If the option to develop the role of the liaison nurse is taken, some changes in the process and structure of the role are indicated to facilitate effective direct liaison between hospital and community nurses.

*Process*

- The development of the liaison role in an advisory capacity. In this way, effective direct hospital nurse–community nurse communication and collaborative discharge planning could be supported.
- To facilitate direct hospital nurse–community nurse liaison, the contribution of liaison nurses to the provision of information about the location of community nurses and community services and facilities.
- The involvement of liaison nurses in encouraging hospital staff to consider the importance of patients' home backgrounds, available community services and the roles of community-based professionals in discharge planning. This could be during formal and informal teaching sessions, at ward meetings, multidisciplinary meetings, ward rounds or on a one-to-one basis.
- The encouragement by liaison nurses to begin discharge planning early during the period of hospitalisation.
- Hospital nurses' accountability for discharge planning needs to be fostered.
- Where appropriate, liaison nurses can involve community nurses in discharge planning.
- Hospital and community nurses, along with other professionals, can be made more aware of the role of liaison nurses by, for example, formal introductory meetings, at the inception of a liaison post, overt management support and continuing educational input from liaison nurses.
- Regular meetings, involving liaison nurses, hospital and community staff allow discussion of any problems experienced with liaison.

## Structure

Where not already evident in the functioning of liaison nurses, the following suggestions for changes would seem useful:

- Liaison nurses need to be experienced community nurses, with relevant experience for involvement with patients needing both district nursing and health visiting follow-up.
- The continuation of funding for liaison posts by community nursing services.
- Liaison nurses should be attached to complete district general hospitals or manageable units of them, rather than to specific client groups, to prevent patients falling through the net.
- The establishment of liaison posts on a full-time and permanent basis.
- The provision of a recognised office base with a telephone for liaison nurses. If possible, an answer-phone and bleep system should be used.
- Formal courses, preparing liaison nurses for their function, are suggested.
- Peer support should be encouraged, both at local and national level. (The Community Nursing Association of the Royal College of Nursing has now developed a Liaison Nurses' Forum.)
- Liaison nurses require more guidance and support on commencing posts, with sufficient flexibility to meet changing organisational needs.

If the option is taken of developing the liaison role as an adviser and educator, positive action needs to be taken to effect change to develop the continuity of patient care.

## References

Amos G (1973) *Care is Rare*. Liverpool: Age Concern.

Armitage S K (1981) Negotiating the discharge of medical patients, *Journal of Advanced Nursing* **6**, 385–9

Armitage S K and Jowett S (1988) *Hospital/Community Liaison Links in Nursing*. Unpublished research report.

Continuing Care Project (1975) *Going Home: The care of elderly patients after discharge from hospital*. Age Concern: Liverpool.

Continuing Care Project (1979) *Organising Aftercare*. London: National Corporation for the Care of Old People.

Continuing Care Project (1980) *Home from Hospital – To What?* (A consultative report). Birmingham: Continuing Care Project.

Donabedian A (1969) Some issues in evaluating the quality of nursing care. *American Journal of Public Health* **59**, 1833–6.

Donabedian A (1980) *Explorations in Quality Assessment and Monitoring*. Volume I: *The Definition of Quality* and *Approaches to its Assessment*. Ann Arbor, MI: Health Administration Press.

Donabedian A (1982) *Explorations in Quality Assessment and Monitoring*. Volume II: *The Criteria and Standards of Quality*. Ann Arbor, MI: Health Administration Press.

Edwards N (1987) *Nursing in the Community: A Team Approach for Wales*. Review of Community Nursing in Wales (Chairman Noreen Edwards). Cardiff: Welsh Office.

Gay P and Pitkeathley J (1978) *When I went Home . . .* London: King Edward Hospital Fund.

Glaser B G and Strauss A L (1967) *The Discovery of Grounded Theory: Strategies for qualitative research*. London: Weidenfeld and Nicolson.

Gordon H (1983) Liaison – the vital link. *Nursing Mirror* **157**, 5, Supplement i–iv.

Jowett S A and Armitage S K (1988) Hospital and community liaison links in nursing: the role of the liaison nurse. *Journal of Advanced Nursing* **13**, 5, 579–87.

Merton R K and Kendall P L (1946) The focused interview. *American Journal of Sociology* **51**, 541–57.

Paxton C M (1974a) Cooperation and care I. *Nursing Times* (Occasional Papers) **70**, 50, 113–6.

Paxton C M (1974b) Cooperation and care II. *Nursing Times* (Occasional Papers) **70**, 51, 117–9.

Reid M and Waddicor P E (1970) Continuity of patient care. *Nursing Times* **66**, 25, 798–9.

Skeet M (1970) *Home from Hospital: A study of the home care needs of recently discharged hospital patients*. London: Dan Mason Nursing Research Committee.

Tuplin J (1984) *The Cost of Liaison and the Role of the Liaison Health Visitor*. London: Unpublished paper, University College Hospital.

Warner V (1981) *Community Nursing Liaison Study* (Preliminary Report). London: Research Unit, Department of Community Medicine, St Mary's Hospital.

Weiss C H (1972) *Evaluation Research – Methods for Assessing Program Effectiveness*. Englewood Cliffs, NJ: Prentice Hall.

# 7
# The Growth and Development of Liaison: A Manager's Perspective

Felicity A Watson

## EDITOR'S INTRODUCTION

Liaison means different things to different people and different ways of working. Felicity Watson describes the evolution of a scheme in which the liaison nurse was initially seen to have an educative role in assisting hospital nurses to establish formal links with community staff. It was thought she would then be able to withdraw! In fact, after an evaluation, her role later developed to an active identification of patients requiring discharge planning. The liaison nurse thus functions in a screening role, with well-defined initial criteria, to determine which patients are likely to require specific discharge planning.

Passing information about known patients in the opposite direction – from community staff to hospital staff – often proves difficult, but is considered essential to adequate discharge planning.

The key point, ensuring the liaison nurse is an integral member of the multidisciplinary team meetings, is central to the success of the scheme. Liaison nursing is viewed not as a stop-gap or isolated individual function but as an element of continuous nursing care which is integral to other parts of the service.

## THE RATIONALE FOR LIAISON

The purpose of a hospital liaison service is to provide suitable communication between hospital and community. From a nurse manager's point of view, the responsibility for developing and supporting such a scheme can give rise to complex problems. Although liaison nurses work in a hospital they are usually responsible to a community manager. Because of the shortage of resources, a liaison service is often provided at the expense of field workers, and this being so, it is essential for such a service to be efficiently managed in order to justify the cost. As with any other member of her staff, the manager is responsible for the recruitment and support of the liaison nurses. The manager should be viewed as a facilitator and resource person to ensure that the liaison nurse can implement the agreed scheme to meet the proposed objectives. However, the nurse manager must be aware of, and be prepared to address, the particular problems that are likely to confront the liaison staff:

1. Liaison nurses will be working in an environment over which their community manager will have no control. Agreement and support for the scheme must be forthcoming from the hospital management, and to this end, close management links must be forged from the outset.
2. Liaison nurses will be working with ward staff who have little concept of the problems faced by patients upon discharge from hospital.
3. The ward staff, often working under the increasing pressures of early discharge and increased patient dependency, have limited time to devote to considering a discharge plan. As a consequence, there is a danger of misusing the liaison nurse when attempts are made to make her responsible for that part of the discharge procedure which should still be the responsibility of the ward staff. The ward staff must retain the responsibility of negotiating the mechanics of the actual discharge with the patient and the patient's carers. This will consist of time and date of discharge, transport arrangements, outpatient follow-up arrangements, together with medicines to accompany the patient and an explanation about drug self-administration.
4. Specialisation has meant that doctors and other health professionals are skilled in one area of medicine at the expense of the holistic approach to care. In acute wards, the management of patients is often seen as management of acute illness or injury, not the longer-term care of disability due to chronic illness.
5. Ward staff have little concept that the role of informal carers is physically, financially and psychologically demanding.
6. Community nurses may already be under the considerable pressure of an increasing workload and although they appreciate the improved planning and communication relating to the discharge of patients they can sometimes view liaison staff in a less than charitable light. Liaison staff are seen to be responsible for the unacceptable increased demands on community nursing time and also have to bear the brunt of criticism when the discharge arrangements are less than satisfactory.

Liaison schemes developed in a haphazard and somewhat disorganised fashion in many general wards and elderly care units in the 1960s and 1970s, and were established to respond to the poor quality of information about discharged patients that was being provided for community nurses; and the increasing number of reports, both research-based and anecdotal, about the poor or total lack of effective discharge planning.

The concept of establishing community-trained nurses in a hospital setting to improve these features of care was essentially new and innovative, and because of this the aims and objectives of this new service were frequently vague and/or flawed.

## STAGE I OF THE SCHEME

It was originally envisaged that the main thrust of the service would be educational, and the role of the liaison nurse would be to:

1. establish formal links between ward and community staff;
2. educate ward staff about the availability of statutory and voluntary services throughout the district, to ensure that effective and efficient use was made of them;
3. formalise and improve the quality of the discharge information being provided to the community nurse.

It was therefore assumed that the task of the liaison nurse would be for a fixed term, following which the ward staff should have developed the necessary skills to be able to plan effectively the discharge of patients.

The multidisciplinary approach which was developing in elderly care units made them an ideal starting point for the scheme. It was found that staff in these areas were enthusiastic about, and interested in, the scope of the service and in some cases already had rudimentary communication systems with the community service.

As the elderly are perhaps the most vulnerable of all patients it was hoped that, by concentrating initially on one unit where liaison was accepted in principle, a working scheme could be developed which could then be used in other areas of the hospital without major modification.

However in acute wards (orthopaedic, surgical, and medical), the reception of the liaison nurse by the ward team may be less positive. Indeed, the whole scheme could be regarded as a major threat as it may be interpreted as an indication of failure in the current discharge planning system. Managerially, it is essential that the aims and objectives of the liaison service are identified and formally established from the outset. They can then be discussed with nursing staff from both hospital and community at both managerial and ward level to ensure that there is a full understanding of the role of the liaison staff. It is an essential and continuing part of the managerial responsibility for the service that evaluation of these aims and objectives occurs.

Considerable opposition to a liaison scheme in acute areas is only to be expected from both medical and nursing staff as it is imagined that the service will interfere with and prolong the existing discharge procedures, culminating in 'blocked beds'. Hospital staff have a preconceived idea that effective planning will take days if not weeks to achieve. For the more disabled patient, they imagine that community services will not be able to provide the necessary level of care and that informal carers may not wish to contribute to this care. It is important that nurse managers from both hospital and community should be closely involved in the early stage of a scheme to support all hospital and community staff, resolve conflicts and thus demonstrate the management backing for the scheme. A high level of diplomacy is required to overcome the potential suspicion and resentment that may meet a new scheme. Nurses are reputedly notorious for their resistance to change. Liaison staff have to work by mutual agreement on other people's wards, and changing negative attitudes can be a long and slow process. In this situation, priority must be given to establishing an effective communication system with the ward staff. Although a patient-oriented service, without cooperation from ward staff, little can be achieved. The ward staff may also be reluctant to give liaison nurses access to patient records. However, it must be explained that the liaison nurses must have access to nursing notes and that they should contribute in writing to these records.

## EVALUATION

The first evaluation of the scheme with which the writer was involved took place after six months (Watson, 1980). Problems of implementation were identified and also some weaknesses in the initial aims and objectives of the scheme. Six points were of particular importance to the future development of the scheme.

### Identifying Patients

It was originally envisaged that ward nurses would identify those patients requiring on-going community support and refer them to the liaison staff.

A review of the service made it apparent that the ward staff had neither the necessary information nor the skills and knowledge of patient care in the community to identify successfully those patients who would require continuing care. Hospital admission and treatment were seen by ward staff as an isolated episode, unrelated to the continuing care process.

## The Needs of Acute Wards

It transpired that contrary to what had been expected at the inception of the liaison scheme, the wards requiring the most time and all the skills of the liaison staff were the acute wards and not the elderly care unit.

In contrast, the elderly care unit, whose staff functioned as a multidisciplinary team, assessed the continuing needs of the patient and family. The establishment of formal links with the community staff and formulation of methods of communication improved the discharge of patients. This was the one area where liaison staff were positively received and their contribution readily accepted and respected. In retrospect, this should have been expected.

The acute wards have many problems which make discharge procedures more complex and, for the patient, potentially hazardous.

- They have a high proportion of elderly patients.
- They frequently do not have a functioning multidisciplinary team with adequate time to assist in the assessment of patients.
- In many ward areas the nursing process has now been accepted as the framework on which nursing care is planned. However, the absence of a nursing model used in conjunction with the nursing process has meant that a holistic approach to care is not always achieved. The focus on problem-solving may have led to a negative view of patients' abilities and skills.
- The average length of a patient's stay, particularly on surgical wards, is frequently short; thus the period of time available in which to undertake discharge planning is very limited.
- Ward staff were extremely over-optimistic in their expectations of the ability of patients and their relatives to cope and did not anticipate many of the difficulties that could occur.
- Ward staff did not appreciate the loss of confidence suffered by patients who had had a prolonged hospital stay.

## Information Sharing

All too often, crucial information which impinged on the process of discharge was not forthcoming from community staff. Liaison nurses were not given initial information on patients who were being visited by community staff prior to admission. Communications with community nurses when patients were admitted required improvement. Community nurses who had visited prior to admission had to be encouraged to relate information to the liaison nurse about the patient, family and environment in which the patient lived. Without this information, given at the time of admission, discharge planning may be ineffective and incomplete. Although community nurses were requested to provide this information of their own volition, the liaison nurses frequently had to be proactive in contacting them. A simple system whereby the community nurse can relay this information should be devised by the community managers and nurses and managers should ensure that this information continues to be forthcoming so that it can properly be considered when patient discharges are planned (Vaughan and Taylor, 1988).

For effective discharge planning to begin, the liaison staff require information in four categories:

1. the condition of the patient prior to admission;
2. the home conditions of the patient;
3. the level of support received (if any) from outside agencies prior to admission;
4. the level of support from informal carers, and their attitude towards continuing care.

## Documentation

For those patients not previously known to the community nursing services, it is essential to document in their nursing record the details of their social circumstances prior to admission. It may be necessary to design a specific record form for this purpose.

## Methods of Communication

The methods of communication used to relay information about discharged patients to community nurses was found to require the following improvements:

1. Information should be in writing and should complement the written nursing record used by the community staff. To avoid duplication of record-keeping, a common nursing record was developed. This form was used by the liaison nurses as a discharge document and also used by the community staff as the basic written record for all community patients. The written information from the liaison staff provided a permanent record of the patient's condition on discharge and would be available to all involved community nurses (see Figures 7.1a and b).
2. Although telephone messages may be necessary on occasion, it was felt important to keep these to a minimum. However, when prompt follow-up by the community nurse was needed, total reliance on any postal system may be unsatisfactory. Telephone information, whenever possible, should be transmitted directly,

HEALTH AUTHORITY: COMMUNITY NURSING RECORD – BASIC INFORMATION

| Surname | Forenames | Title | Address | D.O.B. | Occupation | Religion |
|---|---|---|---|---|---|---|
| | | | | | | Minister/Priest |
| | | | | | | Contact |

| GP Address | District Nurse Address | | Next of Kin 1. Name | | 2. Name | |
|---|---|---|---|---|---|---|
| | | | Address | | Address | |
| Tel. No. | Tel. No | | Tel. No. | | Tel. No. | |

1. Diagnosis

2. Relevant Previous History

3. Date Referred To District Nursing Service

Date Visits Discontinued

Access

Lives Alone

| Hospital Referral Notes | Consultant | Ward | Date of Admission | Date of Discharge |
|---|---|---|---|---|

Summary of Treatment and Conditions on Discharge

Treatment Requested

**Fig. 7.1a   Liaison discharge form/basic community nursing record.**

| Date | Action to be Taken | Observation/Evaluation | Signature |
|---|---|---|---|
|  |  |  |  |
|  |  |  |  |
|  |  |  |  |
|  |  |  |  |
|  |  |  |  |

Fig. 7.1b   Liaison discharge form/basic community nursing record.

nurse to nurse. On occasion, it may be necessary to leave messages with a third party and it must be realised that errors can occur, through misinterpretation by receptionists and clerks who may receive and transmit these referrals.
3. Relevant information should be available to the community nurse prior to the first visit to a patient following discharge from hospital.
4. Many designs of discharge forms have been developed, and in some instances much time spent on refining them. It is important to design a form that is simple and can be used for all discharges. Too much time can be wasted on repeated modification.

## Ward Routine

The liaison staff initially had to develop a good working rapport with the ward staff. Considerable time was required to identify the particular and specific ward routines. It was deemed important that the scheme should complement and not work against the way in which the ward was managed.

## STAGE II OF THE SCHEME

Following evaluation, it was necessary for the manager, together with the liaison and other involved staff, to redefine the aims and objectives of the scheme.

It was questioned whether the scheme should continue to be primarily educational and attempt to provide ward staff with the necessary skills with which to assess need and plan care. Was what was being asked of them an extension of their normal discharge planning procedures?

It was decided that the focus of the scheme should be altered – a change that involved the manager in considerable negotiation and discussion with the staff in both hospital and community settings. Discussion centred on the following points:

1. Community nurses, with the skills learned in community nurse training and practical experience, had the ability to identify more accurately those patients who potentially required continuing care and therefore were most effective in providing a liaison service. Their assessment of patients' actual and potential needs, their expertise in incorporating carers into the planning process and their knowledge of the range and scope of complementary community services were essential to effective planning.

2. The ward-based nurse had little understanding of the interface between informal carers and community nurses. They had an unfounded faith that if patients stated that they could manage (with or without the assistance of carers), this would be the case. If carers of a terminally ill patient stated that they would look after a relative at home, ward staff envisaged that they had the skills to undertake this task and, furthermore, the environment was suitable so that no further referral or planning was necessary.
3. Ward staff had little comprehension of the scope and role of other agencies which were available in the community to provide care and support. They were unable to utilise the full range of local services which could be mobilised at the point of discharge.
4. Ward staff were already working under considerable pressure with the increasing demands of a rapid patient turnover and an accompanying increasing patient dependency. It was difficult to envisage that they would be able to allocate sufficient time to improve their discharge planning effectively.
5. Difficulties over delay in the provision of both services and equipment could not at present be resolved. However, these problems could now be more specifically defined, and communicated to the appropriate agencies.

The aims of the scheme were therefore redefined and the new aims became:

- to improve the discharge planning procedure,
- to improve the quality of information to the community nurse at the point of discharge.

Detailed discharge planning could not be provided for all patients; neither was it necessary. For many patients admitted, for example, for cold surgery the admission had been uneventful, they returned home to supportive families and they had limited need for continuing care. For these patients, the arrangements for post-discharge care were none the less important, but would not be part of the liaison nurse role. It was therefore necessary to develop guidelines to identify patients who would benefit from detailed personalised discharge planning. Selection was made for discharge planning by reviewing the nursing and medical records. The criteria for those requiring discharge planning were:

*The age of a patient*   Those over 65 years were considered to be in need of a home assessment by a community nurse following discharge.
*The diagnosis of a patient*   Patients who were likely to require long-term nursing or who had a high level of dependency were seen to require detailed discharge planning.

*The previous medical history of a patient*  especially underlying long-term illness with or without the provision of community support.
*The social circumstances of a patient*  and in particular the suitability of home conditions for continuing care and both the availability and ability of informal carers.

If it was not immediately apparent from the records that discharge planning was appropriate, patients and their relatives/carers could be consulted about likely problems.

In these circumstances the role of the liaison staff would change so that they worked alongside the hospital staff and assisted them in the following ways (see Figure 7.2):

● by identifying the patients for whom discharge planning was considered necessary, and recording this in the nursing record;

| Liaison Staff | | Ward Staff |
|---|---|---|
| Screening of all patients to identify those in need for discharge planning | ← | Initial patient assessment |
| ↓ | | |
| Additional patient information (previous condition/social circumstances) from community staff | ⇆ | Social circumstances assessment |
| | | ↓ |
| ↓ | | Continuing assessment of patient's physical/psychological condition and care needs |
| Patients/relatives seen to identify potential problems on discharge | | |
| Initial assessment of level of continuing care necessary Nursing equipment | | |
| ↘ | | ↙ |

Joint decisions at case conferences/ward meetings
(All involved Staff)

1. Multidisciplinary patient assessment
2. Patient's suitability to be cared for at home
3. Education needed by patient/carer prior to discharge
4. Support services necessary at home
5. Home visits with patient
6. Equipment
7. Provisional date for discharge

| ↙ | | ↘ |
|---|---|---|
| Patient/relative seen to arrange nursing care. Equipment/information leaflets provided. | → | Routine arrangements for discharge |
| ↓ | | |
| Information communicated to community staff | | |

**Fig. 7.2  Communication flow chart.**

- by devising with nurses and other involved professionals, the patient and relatives/carers, an appropriate discharge plan;
- by liaising with community nurses on the patient's current condition and discussing the potential plans for discharge;
- by assisting with teaching both patients and carers in order to give them confidence to manage appropriate areas of self-care and to enhance independence.

It was necessary to explain the scheme, and subsequently the revised role of the liaison staff, to both hospital managers and ward staff in order to gain their cooperation. It had to be stressed that the liaison role was not one that removed the basic responsibilities for discharge procedures from the ward staff, but one that would enhance their work in effecting satisfactory discharge procedures.

## WORKING WITH OTHER PROFESSIONAL GROUPS

The transition in the role of the liaison staff extended the scope and influence of the scheme. Not only were the liaison staff now working directly with ward nurses but they also became more directly involved with the work of social services staff, occupational therapists and physiotherapists.

As experienced community nurses, the liaison staff were themselves able to decide when a therapist might be beneficial in assessing the patient's ability in matters of daily living. This led to an increase in the number of referrals to the therapists but they accepted the implications of the scheme as a natural extension of their contribution to patient care. They also found the scheme valuable as it gave them the opportunity in sharing their expertise with community nurses who were responsible for much of the continuation and consolidation of the work started by the therapists. The therapist's skill in teaching relatives how to carry out care both safely and effectively proved to be invaluable to nursing staff.

Social workers initially had reservations, however, as they felt that there was considerable overlap with the service they provided. Some social workers were very anxious that relatives would be confused about the respective roles of the social worker *vis-à-vis* the liaison staff.

While recognising and accepting the social workers' concerns, it was undesirable to allow the role of the liaison staff to be defined too specifically, particularly in this developing stage.

Particular emphasis had to be placed on establishing a good communication network with the social workers, and in ensuring that patients and relatives understood the different roles of the social worker and the liaison nurse. The scheme was explained to the social workers and they then appreciated that the liaison nurses would assess all patients and would be instrumental in ensuring appropriate referrals to the social work department. In practice, due to the fact that liaison nurses wore uniform, they were instantly recognisable and their role was easily accepted and understood by patients.

This practice took considerable time to establish and consolidate. Time has shown that there is an overlap of skills in areas such as counselling, support and guidance of carers, and referral to complementary agencies. Many of these such areas had been regarded as primarily the role of the social worker in hospital prior to the development of the liaison service. However, with effective discussion, there is neither duplication nor antagonism between the staff members. This communication network has been developed by direct personal contact, and by working together in ward rounds/ward conferences. Only by personal rapport does this network develop into an effective system.

The liaison staff, having worked previously in a primary health care team setting, were used to the dynamics of team working. They were, however, unused to the size, complexity and lack of coordination of the teams in which they were now functioning.

Each ward had different team members and the level of team cooperation and involvement varied. In some specialties the paramedical and social work staff were well represented and were permanent members of a ward team. In other areas, disciplines other than nursing were poorly represented. Some wards still worked primarily to a model of medical dominance and the idea of community nurse involvement in discharge was an alien one.

Work was also required in discussing the concept of discharge planning with medical staff at all levels from consultant to house officer. The following points had to be emphasised:

- Discharge was no longer to be an abrupt event following a ward round at the conclusion of a patient's treatment.
- Problems relating to discharge were to be identified early in a patient's hospital stay.
- Liaison and other staff were to be given time to resolve problems identified and establish systems of care which could be maintained in the community.

Some of the hospital personnel who were involved prior to discharge were not necessarily seen as part of the team by the ward staff despite having an essential part to play in making discharge planning effective, for example, specialist nurses and appliances personnel. Ward staff often did not understand fully the extensive role of these members of staff. Furthermore, they often did not appreciate the patient's attitude towards health and illness and the time-consuming specialist care that was needed to assist them in coming to terms with disability and loss.

Ward staff, due to the frequently abrupt nature of discharge, had not always arranged for the patient's appliances to be supplied prior to discharge. A lack of appropriate prostheses was shown to cause great distress to patients and frequently resulted in the patient having to make an additional out-patient visit especially for this purpose. Improved communication with earlier involvement of the appliance staff made it possible for the initial prostheses to be provided prior to discharge.

## CONTINUING PROGRESS OF THE SCHEME

After some time, the liaison staff became members of a number of ward teams, although they continually had to work to gain credibility with all members of the team. However, having gained this acceptance, the validity of the team was strengthened by the commencement of weekly multidisciplinary meetings. These were initially modelled by the orthopaedic unit on the system developed in the acute elderly care areas. The idea was discussed by the ward team, including the liaison nurses, as to the potential value of a pre-discharge assessment prior to the consultant's ward round. The medical staff did not become involved in these meetings, but they came to expect that they would be advised of proposed discharge plans at their ward round. Following the success of these meetings other wards were advised of their usefulness and success. By now, other paramedical staff were as supportive of the concepts as were the liaison staff. In these meetings, all patients were discussed and the interchange of ideas became more formalised. Consequently, communication with the patients became much easier and gaining the necessary information from the patient and family proved simpler. The liaison nurse sat with the patient and explained that her role was to try to solve any problems that might occur after discharge from hospital. Patients and relatives were frequently eager to express their worries concerning their longer-term care.

The liaison staff became recognised by the patients as the planners of discharge and it was to them that the question 'when can I go home?' was addressed. A natural development from this has been the request from very ill patients (frequently those who are terminally ill) 'can I go home?'. The liaison nurse was now recognised by patients as well as professional staff as facilitating home care.

The discharge in these circumstances can be achieved very quickly where appropriate. The care such patients may require can present major problems for the community nurses who need to arrange the necessary level of care and equipment required within a very short timespan. It is therefore good practice to involve both specialist nurses and nurse managers in addition to the primary health care team to ensure that appropriate care can be arranged. Although this type of planning is very time-consuming, in the short term it is one of the most valuable patient services as it makes a successful transfer back to community care possible.

Advances in the range of treatments offered to patients have resulted in community nurses having to extend their skills considerably. For example, patients with enteral and parenteral feeding are now frequently discharged to their own home, and children undergoing cytotoxic or antibiotic treatment via long-term intravenous lines can also be nursed at home.

Although it is possible that specialist nurses may be available to visit these patients at home intermittently, it is the community nurse who is expected to provide a more consistent service. The liaison nurse has a unique role in recognising the areas in which patients' care needs are changing and anticipating the additional skills which will be needed by the community nurse. The liaison nurse, in conjunction with her nurse manager, can arrange for appropriate training to be provided for the community nurses. This ensures that they are competent and confident enough to be accountable for their practice, and gain the necessary new skills to enhance home care. Some community nurses may feel reluctant to extend their skills and feel that for such patients home is an unsuitable environment for continuing care, although this is often due to an unfamiliarity with new techniques and a reluctance to become involved with them.

In such circumstances, managerial support can often help to resolve the problems. The nurse managers have a crucial supportive role to play to ensure that antagonism does not occur between the liaison staff and the community staff. However, it is important that community nurses continue to develop and expand their skills to enhance the care of patients within the home environment.

## STATISTICAL INFORMATION

Gathering statistical information can be time-consuming, repetitive and the end-result may not necessarily be useful.

When the liaison service which is described here was commenced it was difficult to anticipate what information would prove useful, hence some changes have been made over the years.

Initially for patients being discharged who required the continuing intervention of community nurses, it was useful to know the total numbers, ages and general practice. Now with the current implementation by the then Department of Health and Social Security (DHSS) of the Körner implementation returns (DHSS, 1987), many health authorities have adopted computer-aided systems for statistical information, some of which include information on patients who have been discharged from hospital. We have therefore been able to review and reduce the need for liaison staff to collate this information.

The statistical information currently recorded is on a diary basis giving daily details of discharged patients. The information refers to:

1. the ward from which the patient was discharged;
2. the name of the patient;
3. the age of the patient;
4. the GP with whom the patient is registered.

From these data, the following information can be obtained:

1. The weekly pattern relating to discharge figures for the whole of the hospital. Mondays and Fridays remain the days on which the largest proportion of patients are discharged.
2. The wards that discharge a high proportion of patients on Friday afternoon and evening. This creates a major problem with patients who subsequently require a first visit by community staff at the weekend.
3. The age of patients being discharged from the acute wards. A high percentage of patients requiring continuing care from these wards are in the 70+ age group.
4. The monthly fluctuations in the number of discharges throughout the year.
5. The total number of patients discharged who require community nurse care.
6. The total number of patients discharged to each practice.

This daily diary system also has the advantage of allowing the liaison staff to deal rapidly with any enquiries relating to a named patient.

## STAFFING OF COMMUNITY NURSE LIAISON SERVICE

Liaison services have developed in a variety of ways throughout the country and it is consequently difficult to specify appropriate staffing levels. It is important to maximise the benefit that liaison nurses can make to discharge planning and for this reason it was decided not to deploy any of the liaison nurses' time either on pre-admission assessments or post-discharge visiting. It was considered that this model of liaison, used primarily in elderly care units and which gave a high level of input to a limited number of individual patients, could not be supported in a rural area. Travelling time would be unacceptably high and the number of patients for whom liaison nurses could effectively provide a service would be limited. It was therefore necessary for pre-admission assessments to be made in one or more of the following ways:

1. by the GP who had requested admission. Local GPs varied in the amount of information they provided both on the patient's medical condition and on the home environment;
2. by other staff, particularly community nurses, who could provide a nursing assessment and diagnosis;
3. by a consultant undertaking a pre-admission domiciliary visit.

Following discharge, the total care of the patient is the immediate responsibility of the primary health care team. Any progress reports on patients after discharge which may be required by hospital professionals can be requested from the community nurse through the liaison staff. These progress reports have a two-fold function:

1. they give hospital staff information on the continuing care and condition of a patient, thus assisting them to see that a hospital stay is part of the continuum of a patient's life;
2. it gives hospital staff an indication of the patient's need for continued hospital support, e.g. attendance at physiotherapy on an out-patient basis, day hospital attendance.

It has been very encouraging to find that the ward staff now frequently request information from liaison nurses on the progress of discharged patients. This demonstrates much more awareness of the problems encountered by the discharged patient.

Liaison time is now allocated to the various units within the district general hospital. The liaison staff work with specific wards and only work outside their patch when another member of staff is on holiday or otherwise absent. One full-time nurse covers the surgical unit: this consists of two wards with 60 beds, one gynaecology ward with 27 beds, the orthopaedic unit of two wards with 60 beds, and the accident and emergency department. The second full-time nurse covers the medical unit: this consists of two wards with 60 beds, the acute elderly care unit of three wards with 60 beds, a chest/ophthalmic ward of 24 beds, and the outpatients' department.

Secondment of liaison staff to specific wards has been regarded as valuable as it provides continuity and understanding of the specific units. This level of commitment gives both members of staff a manageable caseload. Regrettably, it has not been possible to offer a service to three other wards within the district general hospital.

It is essential that the workload is reviewed. An increase in the number of wards covered would have reduced the value of the service to an unacceptable level. The objectives defined in the discharge planning service could not be met and the level of contact with patients, carers and hospital staff would be too brief and ineffectual. It has also been significant to note the hospital ward statistics which show that the total number of discharges has increased in inverse proportion to the average length of stay. Thus the workload of the liaison staff has increased, even though there has been no increase in the number of beds covered. The services offered by the liaison nurses are well accepted and now more extensively used than when established. Their work is valued and their involvement sought at an early stage of a patient's treatment. The staff changes over the years among the liaison nurses have brought new ideas and further development to the service.

The funding for the liaison schemes at their inception came primarily from community unit budgets and, given the expansion of the liaison role, the financial implications of the scheme now require exploring with the budget-holders within the district general hospital.

The financial advantages of an effective liaison scheme, not only to the patient but also to the efficient running of a ward and the community services, have not yet been evaluated.

Given the service, without which many hospital staff state they could not manage, some rationalisation in the source of funding should take place. Some sharing of the cost between hospital and community services must be sought in order to maintain the existing service and, where necessary, to develop and extend it. Accepting the ever-present pressure to make more efficient use of hospital beds by further reducing length of stay and the bed interval time between patients, hospital managers must recognise the need for discharge planning.

## SUPPORT FOR COMMUNITY STAFF WORKING IN A HOSPITAL SETTING

The role of the liaison nurse can be that of a buffer between hospital and community staff. It has been regarded by some as a sinecure, which it most emphatically is not, although it cannot be denied that the job is physically less demanding than that of a community nurse.

The scheme continues to need revision in order to meet changing patient and ward requirements. New staff deployed to the service have brought new ideas and approaches and this is to be encouraged.

**Watch out! There's a problem about**

| Past | Present | Future |
|---|---|---|
| 1. *Medical history*<br>Previous problems<br><br>2. *Social circumstances*<br>Age { Living with elderly relatives?<br>{ Living alone?<br>Type/suitability of housing<br><br>3. *Services* – District nurse<br>– Home care assistant<br>– Meals-on-wheels<br>– Luncheon clubs<br>– Laundry service<br>– Day hospital/Day care<br><br>4. Activities of daily living<br>Personal care<br>Mobility/house bound | 1. Reaction to admission to hospital<br>2. Is the family able to visit?<br>3. Reaction to surgery/treatment<br>4. Early self-management of colostomies/catheters, etc.<br>Are appropriate appliances supplied?<br>5. Counselling needs, e.g. mastectomy patients<br>6. Can patient do activities of daily living independently?<br>7. Does the occupational therapist/physiotherapist/dietitian/social worker need to help?<br>Does the family need to see the doctor to discuss diagnosis/progress/prognosis? | *Planning for discharge*<br>1. *Need for continuing nursing care*<br>Early referral/discussion with community nurse<br>2. *Equipment* – needs to be ordered to arrive *before* discharge<br>3. *Family*<br>What help will the family be able to give. Do they need advice on diet/lifting/transferring/mobility/nursing care?<br>4. *Financial help*, e.g.<br>Attendance allowance<br>Mobility allowance<br>5. *Arrangements for statutory/voluntary help*, e.g.<br>Meals-on-wheels, day hospital, specialist nurses, home care assistants<br>6. *Drugs*<br>Do patients understand about compliance/side-effects, etc.?<br>Can they use 'child-proof' bottle tops? |

**Fig. 7.3   Check-sheet for student nurses.**

Contact between hospital and community managers has also been maintained, and this has led to improved understanding of problems relating to discharge for both parties.

The staff have been encouraged to become involved in the field of education. They are involved in teaching student nurses within the ward setting and they share with the students the stages of planning leading to discharge. The students are then encouraged to visit the patient with the community nurse in order to evaluate the effectiveness of the transfer home. Written information in the form of handouts to remind students of their own responsibilities have also been produced (see Figure 7.3).

Time has also been spent, on a regular basis, with new medical, nursing and paramedical staff to introduce them to the scheme and its objectives. Some trained nursing staff have also had the opportunity of visiting patients at home with a community nurse and have begun to appreciate the problems that returning home can bring for a patient.

The continuing education requirements of the liaison staff themselves have also needed to be addressed. In particular, it has been found that their needs in the field of counselling have been paramount. Spending considerable time, as their work demands, with the chronically sick, the elderly, and the terminally ill, has called for extended skills in this area.

Liaison nurses must also have their knowledge and skills regularly updated with regard to treatments, dressings and specific nursing aspects of continuing care in order to be able to advise their community colleagues.

They often receive verbal reports concerning the progress of patients and, although it is not possible to do so on a routine basis, it is encouraging to the liaison staff to make occasional visits to discharged patients in the community. Particular attention is given to making these visits possible when a terminally ill patient, with whom much planning has been done, has a satisfactory return home and a greatly improved quality of life.

It has also been possible for the liaison staff to visit some of the peripheral hospitals and social services residential homes which has been particularly helpful in assisting patients to come to terms with the fact that they can no longer manage at home.

## CONCLUSION

At present, liaison staff have only the responsibility of planning discharge. Although it has been debated many times, the onus for discharge in acute hospitals remains with the medical staff and although the liaison staff may be instrumental in delaying discharge, they can rarely prevent it. The community nursing services are currently trying to accommodate the increasing demands, not only from a rising number of discharged hospital patients, but also the increasing number of elderly people in the community and the emphasis on community care. The increase in day surgery, the reducing average length of hospital stay and the realisation that long-term high-tech nursing can be carried out at home have all led to an expectation by medical staff that the follow-up care can and will be forthcoming. The liaison nurse with responsibilities to both hospital and community staff may have to bring influence to bear, not only on the discharge planning, but also on fuller pre-admission assessment and on the possibilities and impossibilities of continuing care at home. Her role may alter to effect these changes and to ensure that the planning with patients is done with an assurance that once at home, the necessary care will be provided. The liaison staff should also be instrumental in suggesting and supporting alternative sources of help, particularly in the field of voluntary services, which may assist in patient discharge.

From a management point of view, despite the complex and demanding nature of the liaison role, it is essential that the staff are adequately supported to ensure that they can carry out their work without excessive demands and frustrations.

Effective, efficient transfer from hospital to home is dependent on the interplay between many different sections of health care and relies on a good communication system. A well-run scheme does much to enhance the patient's well-being and the carer's confidence and this is the positive aspect of the liaison role which must be strongly projected at all times.

## References

DHSS (1987) *Korner Implementation.* Statement of Central Requirements for Aggregated Returns on Community Health Services. London: HMSO.

Vaughan B and Taylor K (1988) Homeward bound. *Nursing Times* **84,** 15, 28–31.

Watson F A (1980) 'Evaluation of Liaison Services at the West Cumberland Hospital', unpublished.

# 8
# Shortening the Information Chain
### Denise E Barnett

## EDITOR'S INTRODUCTION

On many occasions when the intention is to improve the continuity of nursing care additional documentation is introduced which sum- marises the main points relating to a patient's stay in hospital and which is then passed to the community nurses. Nursing process has been with us in concept since the mid-1970s with the assessment of each patient's individual need for the most appropriate care. Entailed in its systematic approach to nursing care is the final stage of evaluation; one which is often largely ignored by nurses.

Denise Barnett describes a project which combined her work on developing patient care plans and within that the evaluative stage of the process with the communication of information to district nurses at the time of a patient's transfer from hospital to home.

An unwritten intention of the project was to build bridges between nurses working within the two settings of hospital and community. The use of evaluation of nursing process as a line of communication to district nurses is demonstrated as an active element which can better enable continuing care to be realised.

## BACKGROUND TO THE RESEARCH PROJECT

Why is it that when the communication chain fails, nurses wish to add another link to it in the form of a liaison nurse? The district nurses in Tower Hamlets who carried out liaison did so with the intention of educating their hospital colleagues about the requirements of the patient within the community. They visited specific wards once each week to discuss planned transfers. Information was then passed on to the relevant community nurse who was attached to a general prac- tice or formed part of the team providing primary health care for a defined geographical area or neighbourhood. In 1976 a very detailed set of guidelines entitled 'Discharge to Community Care' was put together by the then Senior Nursing Officer for Hospital/Community

Liaison (Corkhill, 1976). The transfer form linked to these guidelines was brief and task-oriented. It no longer fitted the developing use of systematic, individualised patient care entailed in the nursing process.

As the Director of Clinical Nursing Research for the health district I was involved in carrying out research projects and in assisting colleagues to investigate their own practice. Some nurses have a preconceived view of the nurse involved in research. It is assumed that research is only about academic interests and therefore the results are not expected to have practical value. Having continued to maintain clinical practice skills throughout my career, I was keen to provide tools and systems which would be of practical use in caring for patients.

For the first two years in this post my work was mainly on the development of an easy to use method of recording nursing care plans and in introducing the nursing process in a variety of wards. The care plan design developed steadily in response to the comments from staff. Five papers outlining this and the associated research were published in a monthly *Nursing Times* series and as a set of papers (Barnett, 1982). Working alongside nurses and students in caring for patients provided many insights into the difficulties of communication and the transition from a task-oriented approach to a patient-centred one (RCN, 1986).

There seems to be a change in self-image when a nurse moves into community nursing. This may well have its roots in the former scheme of management by the local authority rather than the hospital service. Integration of the two components of the National Health Service in 1974 brought with it many opportunities. However, although the integration of nurses into one service has been achieved in many superficial ways, it has been slow to develop on an emotional level. Building bridges between nurses who think of themselves primarily as 'community nurses' or 'hospital nurses', rather than nurses who happen to work in different settings, was one of my unspoken objectives.

A three-year research project to evaluate the effect of nursing care plans on the care actually received by patients required the introduction of a system to aid nurses to develop the evaluation process. Other research workers in the health district had been investigating the problems of ensuring continuity of care on transfer of the patient to the community. In addition, the district nurses had expressed disquiet with the current system and it was therefore opportune to integrate the evaluation of nursing care at the end of a patient's stay with a new transfer letter. It was hoped that by sharing the ward nurse's detailed evaluation of the changes in the patient's problems with the community nurses, a better understanding of each other's role might develop. In addition, the ward nurses needed more detailed feedback from the community staff on the efficiency of the transfer of patients between hospital and community.

## KEY FEATURES IN THE DESIGN OF THE THREE-PART NURSING CARE PLAN FORM

The care plan designed for use in the first part of the research had a flowchart format (see Figure 8.1). This was to meet the ward sisters' perceived need of an at-a-glance view of the patient's problems and the nursing care required that day. The emphasis of the nursing care prescription was on precise actions to be carried out by the nurse rather than generalised statements of intent. The heading of 'nursing action' was therefore used.

Earlier work in the district's hospitals by Hunt and Marks-Maran (1980) had introduced the use of problem statements and descriptions of outcome. The first part of the research had emphasised the description of the problem as it affected the individual patient, using objective measures whenever possible so that change could be detected by a nurse not present during the initial assessment. For 'at-a-glance' use, these descriptions had to be short, pithy and to the point. Small boxes on the form were used to encourage this.

A similar brief description of the desired outcome was to be recorded alongside the problem box. For the new project the lower part of each box was divided to hold the review frequency and evaluation frequency for the problem.

These terms need a little explanation. I had been fortunate in winning a scholarship to visit three centres of excellence in the US to examine their methods of achieving the evaluation stage of the nursing process cycle. I returned with the impression that descriptions in their books and journals were found not to be useful in practice. The theory was only partially translated into action and written evaluations did not seem to reflect changes in the care plan.

Contacts in England and Wales confirmed that nurses were having difficulty with the evaluation stage of the process cycle. It seemed that the difficulty stemmed from the assumption that any nursing action produced immediate observable change in the patient. Clinical experience convinced me that this was not always the case. Certain nursing actions had to be repeated at regular intervals before observable change occurred, an example being oral hygiene for the patient arriving with a caked, dry, dirty mouth. Oral hygiene procedures needed to be carried out every hour or more frequently for some time before any measurable change was apparent and thus

Name ......... Mr. Freddy Smith .........

HEALTH AUTHORITY

| Date | Patient's Problems | Goals/Outcome | NURSING ACTION Date 11/6/85 | Date 12/6 | Date 13/6 | Date 16/6 | Date 20/6 |
|---|---|---|---|---|---|---|---|
| 11/6/85 | Reluctant to get out of a chair and walk following a fall 10/6 | Able to walk with stick at least 4m (distance to loo at home). Review: Daily at 20°° Evaluation: Weds. **1A** | 1. Provide stick 2. Two nurses to support him 3. Walk out to toilet every hour 09°°-19°° 4. Physio | → | → To Dept 10°° each day | To use stick, 1 nurse to support, 1 to walk on left side → | 1 nurse to walk on left. Walk to toilet every 2 hours → |
| 11/6/85 | Has been neglecting his personal hygiene, fine finger movements limited so leaves buttons undone | No body odour. Looks clean and neatly dressed. Review: 14.°° hrs Evaluation: Mon **1B** | 1. 'Argo' bath with 2 staff to help 2. Ask son to review clothes at home | 1. Assisted wash at basin — assess dexterity. | 1. Bath alt days / wash at basin 2. Help him dress — can put on jumper/vest socks/pants → | assist with trousers → | → |
| 11/6/85 | Incontinent of urine as he can't reach the loo in time or unbutton his flies | Able to reach toilet in time and undo flies (see 1a). Review: 08°° + 20°° Evaluation: Wed **1C** | 1. Pyjama parts until son can fetch 2 prs trousers for Velcro adaptation | | → Volunteer will remove buttons and sew on 'Velcro' → | Teach him how to use Velcro fastenings → | |
| 11/6/85 | Bruised and painful left hip following fall yesterday | Feels pain is controlled. Review: 08°° 14°° 20°° Evaluation: Wed **1D** | 1. Paracetamol as prescribed 2. Bed cradle at night | → | → | Solved 18-9-85 → | |
| 11/6/85 | Deaf in LEFT ear, reluctant to wear his hearing aid, RIGHT ear - fair | Can understand and join in conversation. Review: 14.°° hr Evaluation: Tues **1E** | 1. Hearing aid will be fetched from home by son 2. Speak slowly in his right ear | → | Hearing aid sent for repair → | → | To wear aid for morning - unused to background noise |

Fig. 8.1 Nursing care plan

before the response to the procedure could be assessed. It would only be at this point that a partial judgement on the effect could be made and the frequency amended or confirmed as adequate to achieve the desired level of improvement. However, with a different nurse on each of three shifts such partial judgement required a written record so that incremental changes could be considered when reassessing the appropriateness of the prescribed care. These descriptions of change were named 'reviews'.

The evaluation of the plan and the degree of response achieved was then undertaken at longer intervals and work in the acute wards indicated that once a week was a useful starting point. As nurses became used to recording descriptions of the patient's response in measurable terms and in linking these to the problem identification code, evaluations became relatively quick and easy to do. It was hoped that in time the frequency of evaluation would be set for each problem rather than all those recorded on the form.

Reliance on a large proportion of students rather than qualified nursing staff in hospitals had resulted in little use of any in-depth knowledge. The quality of information collected and transmitted to community nurses was poor and task-oriented. This was slowly changing as the systematic approach to nursing began to reveal the gaps in knowledge among not only student nurses but also qualified staff. The gaps in students' knowledge were hardly surprising. Qualified nurses were unaware of research findings so that it was hardly likely that students would see them put into practice in planning care. Over the period of the research action was taken to begin to redress the imbalance between the proportion of students and qualified staff.

The opportunity was taken to emphasise the amount of nursing knowledge needed to evaluate the effect of planned nursing action on the progress of patients and the outcome achieved by the date of transfer. Evaluation was seen as an activity to be carried out by a qualified nurse; thus if the record was to be shared with the district nurse the communication would be between qualified nurses. The corollary of this was that it was inappropriate for a hospital nurse to instruct a colleague in another specialist field on how to nurse a patient. Instead, suggestions for further action would be made. Information would then be provided to add to the results of the community nurses' assessment so that a new care plan could be prepared for use in the patient's home.

In line with the move towards sharing more information with colleagues came the desire to share more with the patient. District nurses and their managers began to discuss how best to inform and involve patients in decisions about nursing care. It was agreed to redesign the community nursing records so that they could be left in the patient's home for reference by the patient, his or her carers and by fellow professionals. The working group, of which I was a member, redesigned the initial assessment forms and the progress sheets. A folder with six filing points was used to hold in order of appearance: the list of medications taken by the patient, the referral letter(s), the assessment sheets (four sides of general assessment and four in-depth assessments for specific problems), the care plan sheets (which could display up to 10 problems) the progress and evaluation notes, correspondence, and finally, on the back cover, a log of each home visit. The front of the file included the patient's name and address together with information about how to contact the nurse and details about any other professionals visiting the patient.

## LOCAL PROBLEMS IN THE DISCHARGE PROCESS

A group of hospital and community nurses agreed to advise on the content of the general information which a hospital nurse could transfer to community colleagues. It was agreed that the integration of the nursing service should be emphasised by using the term 'transfer' rather than the commoner 'discharge' to the community.

During the development of a new form to convey information from hospital to the community nursing service a number of points were taken into account.

Regular complaints from the district nurses included the following:

- The discharge address was sometimes incomplete or inaccurate. This led to time wasted in searching and worries for the patient when the nurse did not visit as expected.
- Elderly people were reluctant to open the door to strangers and, unless some form of identification had been agreed, access was sometimes very difficult. Ward staff failed to appreciate this and also failed to arrange with the immobile patient and the district nurse the location of the house key so the nurse could let herself in.
- Ward staff failed to include details of how much the patient could undertake unaided and the involvement of carers so that patients sometimes relapsed into dependence.
- Ward staff also failed to convey what diagnosis had been given to the patient and relatives and also the likely prognosis. This led to wary verbal 'play' around the topic until the district nurse was able to discuss the situation with the GP. As the letter from the hospital doctor was sometimes delayed, this could mean quite a time-lag before the nurse felt confident to answer questions.

A questionnaire focusing on these points was developed to accompany the new summary/transfer information. The district nurse's opinion was also sought on the usefulness of the information about each problem and whether the proposed nursing action could be carried out at home.

An analysis of the number of patients transferred to the district's community nurses showed that the geriatric assessment ward provided a steady flow. Other wards transferred one or two patients a week and would therefore not achieve a large enough sample without markedly extending the period of the project. The ward staff were interested in participating and the liaison district nurse had an interest in developing the use of the nursing process.

## DESCRIPTION OF THE RESEARCH PROJECT IN A GERIATRIC ASSESSMENT WARD

### General Preparation

A number of small details consumed considerable time and effort, as they tend to do in a financially hard-pressed health district. To supply the geriatric ward with relevant stationery took several weeks for the Director of Nursing Services (DNS) to identify funding for 500 sets of the forms. A second problem was postage. It was essential that information was transferred to the community nurse prior to the patient's discharge. The internal mail distribution system had repeatedly proved too slow, material being delivered 3-4 days *after* a patient had returned home. The alternative use of first class mail generated considerable discussion, mainly because of the cost. In the geriatric assessment ward the policy was to try to arrange for patients to go home on Tuesday, Wednesday or Thursday to give time for unsatisfactory services to be corrected before the weekend. This meant that lack of mail collection and delivery on a Sunday was not a problem. Eventually the DNS was able to persuade the unit administrator to agree to the extra expense of first class stamps.

### Introducing Review and Evaluation Techniques

Care plans had been well established in the ward before the project began but the evaluation of nursing care was not. The admission assessment might be undertaken by a qualified nurse or by a student nurse who would then discuss the observations with a qualified nurse. The care plan based on the assessment might be prepared by either. Patients were allocated to learners on a geographical basis. However, in the geriatric assessment ward the day room was used for a large part of the patients' day. One student would be allocated to work with patients in the day room while colleagues assisted their allocated patients with washing and dressing.

The written reports were still typical of the old style 'Kardex'. It was necessary to introduce new ideas about describing the patient's response to nursing action for specific problems and for regular evaluation of the influence of the planned care on the patient's response.

The intention was that each care plan form would be numbered sequentially and the sheet number inserted beside the printed letter in the problem box (A–E) to provide a code for each problem. This was then used in the progress notes beside the description of the patient's response to nursing action. The frequency of these descriptions or reviews was prescribed in the care plan to guide the student as to how often to make a written record. In long-stay wards for the elderly, it was agreed that some nursing auxiliaries could also record review information.

The evaluation could focus on the effects of:

- nursing actions on a single problem;
- nursing actions on all the problems of one patient;
- the available resources, or lack of them, on care;
- ward, nursing, medical or hospital policies on nursing care;
- the knowledge and skills of the individual nurse on care;
- specific teaching or education on nursing action and its prescription.

In addition, the weekly evaluation aimed to summarise the degree of change in the patient's condition during the preceding week and to comment on any alteration in the expected rate of change together with the likely reason. Limitations on the available resources, particularly in the amount of nursing time to meet the identified patient's needs, provided useful evidence for nurse managers of understaffing and its effects on patients. During the same session, if the nurses evaluated the care planned for several problems, then interrelationships might be identified. Discussion sometimes revealed new problems or new courses of action which were then added to the care plan.

At the end of the patient's stay in hospital these weekly evaluations were to be summarised and an evaluation made of the degree of change achieved since the problem was first identified. A brief description of the current state of any continuing problem was to be added as a starting point for the community nurse. For an example of a summary/evaluation form completed for a fictitious patient see Figure 8.2.

HEALTH AUTHORITY

Name: Mr. Freddy Smith

| Date | Patient's Problems | Goals/Outcome | SUMMARY OF ACTION AND CURRENT STATE OF PROBLEMS (If resolved give date of resolution) | SUGGESTIONS FOR FURTHER ACTION ON TRANSFER |
|---|---|---|---|---|
| 11/6/85 | Reluctant to get out of a chair and walk following a fall 10/6. 1A | Able to walk with stick at least 4m (distance to loo at home). Review: Daily at 20:00h Evaluation: Weds | Initially needed 2 nurses to support him, tended to lean to the left and was unsteady. Little confidence at first. Daily physio in Dept. from 13/6 to 23/6. Now walks with stick unsupported, prefers someone with him. Can walk 8m at a time. | He may feel move confident in his own home with furniture for support. Home assessment required. |
| 11/6/85 | Has been neglecting his personal hygiene, fine finger movements limited so leaves buttons undone. 1B | No body odour. Looks clean and neatly dressed. Review: 14:00 hrs Evaluation: Mon | Alternate days bath and wash at basin until 22/6 then bath every 4th day. Reluctant to wash more than his face and hands until 21/6. Still unsteady when he reaches for feet. Will need supervision for some time yet. Can wash unaided at basin. | Visit from nursing auxiliary midweek for bath, son will help him each weekend. Needs chair kept by washbasin. Can dress unaided if no buttons. Elastic shoe laces. |
| 11/6/85 | Incontinent of urine as he can't reach the loo in time or unbutton his flies 1C | Able to reach toilet in time and undo flies (see 1a). Review: 08:00 + 20:00h Evaluation: Wed | Walked to toilet hourly 05:00 → 19:00 until 20/6 then 2 hrly, 3 hrly from 27/6. Continent by day, uses urinal in bed at night. Velcro instead of fly buttons a great success! | Son has purchased urinal for use at home. See 1A. |
| 11/6/85 | Bruised and painful left hip following fall yesterday 1D | Feels pain is controlled. Review: 08:00, 14:00, 20:00 Evaluation: Tues | Paracetamol given 4 hrly until 13/6. Then as required – 2 doses 14/6, 1 dose at night 15, 16, 17/6. Not required after 18/6. Bed cradle until 16/6. Bruise faded slowly as pain subsided. Problem solved 18/6/85 | |
| 11/6/85 | Deaf in LEFT ear, reluctant to wear his hearing aid, RIGHT ear-fair. 1E | Can understand and join in conversation. Review: 14:00 hr Evaluation: Tues | Hearing aid was chipped and tube split. Repaired 16/6. Wearing times built up slowly. Tends to want TV/radio on rather too loud for others' comfort. Now quite a chatterbox! | Loop-induction system for ? Light to replace doorbell. Appt. at Hearing Aid Clinic 10/7/85. Would appreciate visits from volunteers? Church Group. |
| | Evaluation Completed By I. M. Harte | | Grade: Staff Nurse on: 4/7/85 | COMMUNITY COPY |

Fig. 8.2 Summary/evaluation of nursing care.

| | | |
|---|---|---|
| Hospital  Anytown | Ward  5A | Record No  000001 |

**\*Consultant**  Dr Snoddy                    **Date of discharge**

**Name**  Mr Freddy Smith

**Home Address**  123 The Avenue, Anytown

**Length of anticipated stay at Discharge Address**  ———

**Special points for community staff to gain access** (e.g. who holds a key or what is agreed code of knocks on door to identify nurse, deafness, slow to walk to door etc.)  Deaf if he is not wearing hearing aid. Walks slowly with a stick. Key left at No 124 (Mrs Brown)

| | | |
|---|---|---|
| **\*Date of Birth**  2/2/07 | **\*Age**  78 | **\*Religion**  C/E |

**Marital Status**  widower (last 7 years)          **\*Lives: Alone** / ~~With Spouse~~ / ~~With Friend or Relative~~

| | | |
|---|---|---|
| **\*Next of Kin**  Mr Mathew Smith | **\*Relationship to Patient**  Son |

**\*Address**  4 The High Street
            Seatown

**\*Telephone Number**  111 0004

**Information about diagnosis** ~~and/or prognosis~~ **given to patient and/or Next of Kin**  Simple anaemia (Hb 9.2 on admission) due to poor diet. Now Hb 10.6, on oral iron — see letter to G.P. OPD Appt in 10/52 (will be sent on)

**Neighbours, friends or other relatives involved in the care of the patient**  Son lives 25 miles away — will visit each Sunday to bath Freddy

**\*General Practitioner**  Dr P Greene

**\*Address**          The Surgery
            Anytown

**\*Telephone Number**  111 0019

**Services already organised from Hospital but not included in the Nursing information overleaf**

Home help requested

Meals on wheels Mon → Friday (may manage Luncheon Club visits soon)

| | | | |
|---|---|---|---|
| **Information Prepared By**  I. M. Harte | **Grade** Staff Nurse | **on**  4/7/85 | 198— |

**Fig. 8.3 Information from hospital to community nursing service.**

In this way the district nurse would be provided with an overview of the patient's stay in nursing terms. An additional column provided space for the hospital nurse to suggest further action for unresolved problems. General information was provided on the back of the sheet, see Figure 8.3.

## Preparation of Staff

Teaching sessions were held for registered and enrolled nurses. Times were agreed and the researcher went to the ward to work with one or two members of staff at a time. The ward seminar room was used and sessions were interrupted by patients wandering in or by staff being called out into the ward to deal with problems. Some sessions were cancelled at short notice because of changes in the ward workload. Similar problems were experienced in earlier projects in the district and reported by Ashworth (1984) in Manchester. For this project the Christmas period with all its attendant parties and entertainments for the patients also reduced the amount of available time for teaching sessions.

Staff worked in pairs to prepare a weekly evaluation of care for one or two patients. As they became more comfortable with the new approach the number of patients considered in each session increased. In an acute ward a weekly evaluation of the whole care plan was suggested. In long-stay wards the interval might be 4–6 weeks. Some of the patients in the acute wards were awaiting places in the long-stay wards. It was agreed that weekly evaluations would be carried out during the acute phase of illness and then the frequency would decrease as the pace of the patient's response to rehabilitation altered, thus the overall workload was reduced. The weekday on which a patient's evaluation would be carried out was recorded in the care plan. The evaluation workload was thus spread out through the week. The design of the care plan form was flexible enough for different frequencies of evaluation to be set for problems. For example, some elderly patients had chronic deficits such as deafness or poor vision, for which nursing action was required such as battery checks on the hearing aid or an illuminated magnifying glass. The planned nursing action for these problems might be evaluated every 2–3 weeks, while the acute problems for which the patient had been admitted would be evaluated weekly.

Once the staff felt confident in their weekly evaluations, a summary/evaluation of the whole of the patient's stay was prepared prior to discharge and placed in a wallet file in the ward. The researcher collected these at intervals and, using red ink, annotated the comments to indicate to ward staff those areas not covered that might be helpful to a community nurse. It was important for the ward staff to feel confident about the quality of the summary before exposing their efforts to the critical eyes of community colleagues. It was anticipated that some of the district nurses might find the changes hard to accept and the ward staff would need to be able to cope with any negative comments. Developing something new is always risky and nurses tend to have firm views on the correct ways of doing things.

The ward sister also identified a problem among the night staff who were not directly involved in the weekly evaluations or the summary/evaluations and who continued to use the traditional stylised entries in the progress notes which made some evaluations difficult. The researcher arranged to provide teaching sessions at 23.00 hours for the night sisters and charge nurses who needed extra help and support to develop the use of progress notes.

The interest and involvement of most of the staff was impressive, particularly as the ward was always busy. Especially at the beginning of this project staff sometimes stayed on duty at the end of a shift in order to complete evaluations of patient care.

## Preparing for Data Collection

It was agreed to set a date after which all patients newly admitted would have their care plans recorded on the new three-part forms. This gave a period of several weeks before likely transfers and the need to pass information to community colleagues. The chosen date was 20 January 1985 and the first forms were issued on 15 March. The yellow ward copy was to be placed in a folder for collection by the researcher. If this was done once a week, it would mean that the copy would be available for reference in the ward for a few days after transfer.

The district nurses were advised through their nurse managers that new pink summary/evaluation sheets were now in use by the ward and that their cooperation in completing the associated questionnaire would be appreciated.

The ward was supplied with numbered sets of envelope, explanatory letter, questionnaire and return envelope addressed to the researcher. A log sheet with the same numbering system was left inside the folder. The ward nurse was asked to include a questionnaire with the patient's summary/evaluation and to add a return date of three weeks hence in the space provided at the end of the questionnaire. The patient's name and date of transfer was then to be added to the log sheet beside the relevant code number. The ward nurse addressed the envelope to the appropriate community nurse using the district list of GP practices and their attached/related community staff. No record was kept of the name of the community nurse to whom the questionnaire was sent so that all replies were anonymous.

## COMPARISON OF WARD AND DISTRICT NURSE'S VIEWS OF THE SAMPLE PATIENT TRANSFERS

The first six pairs of summary/evaluation sheets and questionnaires had to be excluded from the study as the ward nurses had not completed the sections for the summary and suggested further action. This omission was fed back to the ward team.

The next sixteen logged questionnaires and evaluation summaries were sent out between 20 March and 30 April 1985. Twelve completed questionnaires were returned to the researcher (75 per cent response rate). A further 28 questionnaires were sent out between May and the end of June. The overall response rate for the study was 59 per cent.

### Access and Discharge Address Information

The first two questions of the questionnaire were linked:

1. Was the information on the form about the access and the address to which the patient was discharged sufficient for your first visit?
2. If the information was *not* sufficient please explain briefly:
   (a) what, if anything, was missing
   (b) what, if anything, was incorrect
   (c) what difficulties (if any) did this cause?

The district nurses reported that the discharge address was inaccurate for five patients and incomplete for one. The omission of the number of the patient's flat gave one district nurse problems. She rang the bottom bell to be answered by an annoyed tenant who had been resting. Mrs P lived in the top flat and could only make her way very slowly down to the front door. This information had also been omitted so that the nurse had given up waiting and left by the time the patient reached the door.

In another instance the wrong address was given and the district nurse had to obtain the correct one from the patient's neighbours. Another nurse's time was wasted looking for an address with the wrong post code and for the wrong block of flats. With patients known to the community nursing service problems were avoided because of prior knowledge.

For one lady the discharge information was incomplete, although this was not entirely the fault of the ward nurse. The family had discussed their plans with the ward doctor who had failed to mention them to the staff. Mrs B was collected from her home each day by one of her daughters, spent the day with her and was then taken back to her own home for the night. The district nurse could not obtain a reply when calling at the patient's house. She tried to telephone one daughter but could get no reply so she phoned the ward staff who were equally puzzled. It took a week before the mystery was solved and the patient seen by the district nurse.

## Information about Neighbours, Friends or Relatives

District nurses were asked to comment on whether the information about neighbours, friends and relatives was useful (7 responses), already known (10), accurate (2), incomplete (2) or incorrect (3). Of the two incomplete items of information, one concerned the absence of a resident warden and the relief warden was not present when the patient was transferred home. Local wardens were usually very helpful in visiting their elderly residents and in assisting the old person to settle in on transfer from hospital. The other problem concerned the address of a patient's son whose brother was given as the next of kin. There was no mention of the son and his address. The patient refused to let the nurse in unless her son was present. It was only on the third day that the district nurse gained access to the patient.

The three incorrect items were the inability of Mr A's wife to cope with his care, the already mentioned daily movement of Mrs B to her daughter's flat and lack of available care for Mrs H whose sister lived upstairs, had a telephone and could cope with washing, dressing and weekend meals. The district nurse suggested that Mrs H may have told the ward nurses that no one was involved in her care.

Problems were also caused by the omission of details of Mrs C's neighbour's holiday arrangements. Prior to Mrs C's admission her neighbour had cared for her each day but was still away when Mrs C went home so that there was no one to check on her well-being.

## Support Services

District nurses were asked to indicate whether the following services had been requested by the hospital, and if so whether they had arrived as expected: home help, meals-on-wheels, chiropody and visits from a social worker or health visitor. Other services requested included help with bathing, twilight nursing service and a visit by the diabetic liaison nurse (see Table 8.1).

Table 8.1   Support Services

| Result | Home help | Meals-on-wheels | Chiropody | Diabetic liaison | Bathing | Twilight nursing | Day centre |
|---|---|---|---|---|---|---|---|
| Requested and received | 8 | 8 | 1 | 1 | 2 | 2 | 1 |
| Awaiting assessment | 1 | | | | | | |
| Not arrived | 1 | | | 1 | | | |
| Arrived or not | 3 | | | | | | |
| District nurse request | | 1 | | | | | |
| Incomplete answer | | | 1 | 2 | | 1 | |
| Total number of patients | 13 | 9 | 2 | 4 | 2 | 3 | 1 |

No visits from the social worker or health visitor had been requested for the 44 patients included in the study. This lack of referral in a group where 34 of the patients were considered by either hospital or community staff to require one or more services is interesting. Gooch (1988) suggests health visitors may be considered too precious a commodity to waste on work with the elderly. An alternative view may be that the district nurse would include the same assessment as the health visitor, so that only one referral was necessary.

Home help had been requested for 13 patients, one of whom was still awaiting assessment. The service had not arrived for another and for three patients no comment was made as to whether the service had arrived or not. The others had received the service as expected.

Meals-on-wheels had been requested by the hospital for eight patients and the district nurse had put in a request for the ninth. The latter produced considerable delay which could have been avoided had the ward staff realised that, without neighbours or friends, assistance would be required.

Chiropody had arrived as expected for one patient, and the district nurse's answer for a second patient was incomplete.

The diabetic liaison nurse had called on one patient but not the second one. There were incomplete answers for another two.

Help with bathing had arrived as expected for the two patients for whom it was requested.

The twilight nursing service had visited two patients for whom it was requested. The answer for the third was incomplete.

Day care attendance had been successfully arranged for one patient.

**Care Plan Content**

There were 24 sets of care plans which could be married up with the completed questionnaires by their code numbers. These consisted of 114 problems identified during the patient's admission with 2–10 problems per patient (median 4.5). The problem descriptions varied in length and detail but could be grouped into the following, representing 91 problem themes:

- disordered mental state (including confusion, depression, disorientation and anxiety) [16];
- reduced mobility (including walking and use of hands) [12];
- difficulty in maintaining personal hygiene [11];
- loss of appetite [10];
- urinary frequency and incontinence [9];
- risk/presence of pressure sores [8];
- leg ulcers and other lesions [7];
- diabetes mellitus [6];
- constipation and diarrhoea [5];
- dehydration [3];
- lethargy or drowsiness [2];
- abdominal discomfort [2];

Of the 114 problems, 49 were known about by district nurses and action at home was required for 54 problems.

Only seven of the problems identified in hospital and still current were considered no longer to be a problem in the home. They involved three patients and are given verbatim to illustrate some of the difficulties in interpretation which may face the district nurse:

| Problem | Summary/Evaluation |
| --- | --- |
| 1. Unable to maintain her own personal hygiene | Washes and dresses with minimal assistance. Will possibly need help most mornings. |
| At risk of pressure sores due to immobility. | Mobilises independently, but needs help to get up. Uses a frame. *Unsigned* |
| 2. Congestive cardiac failure | Still remains breathless but is able to cope, gets weary easily. |
| Deafness | Is still deaf. |
| Tendency to be unsteady on her feet | Walks well with her stick *Registered Nurse* |

| | |
|---|---|
| 3. Abdominal discomfort | Barrier [sic] meal carried out; no abnormal findings. Pain has been control [sic] with analgesia Paracetamol as per required. Medical staff think that pain is due to psychosomatic cause. |
| Drowsiness and loss of energy | Still very lethargic and lacking in energy; has been adviced [sic] to rest in between meals and lay down if she feels very exhausted. *Student Nurse* |

The third example, prepared by the student nurse, illustrates the difficulties that can accompany poor grammar and spelling and lack of understanding of the treatment by those in hospital providing care.

Four problems known to the district nurse had been resolved by the hospital, and a further two present on admission had been solved during the hospital stay. There was no comment from the district nurses on 14 problems.

As the questionnaire had omitted to ask whether the patient was known to the district nursing service prior to admission it was difficult to comment on the significance of unresolved problems recognised by hospital and community nurses. The geriatric assessment ward had a section for elderly people with possible mental illness and the proportion of patients in the category of 'disordered mental state' may reflect this. It may also be an indication of which patients were referred to the district nurse.

### Nature of the Summary/Evaluation Comments (See Table 8.2)

During the preparatory teaching the researcher fed back to the ward staff the nature of their comments made in the trial forms. Missing information was highlighted. The copies of the care plans were analysed to see whether the three desired components were present for every current problem. These were:

- summary of the action taken;
- description of the patient's response;
- description of the current state of the problem.

Only four of the 106 current problems had all three components.

The most frequent component was the description of the current state of the problem (54) with some including words such as 'remains' (15) or 'still' (10) to indicate that the patient's condition had been maintained.

**Table 8.2  Summary/evaluation comments**

Number of problems categorised by nature of comments in the summary/evaluation section of the forms.

| | | |
|---|---|---|
| Resolved | | 8 |
| Action summary | (A) | 7 |
| Response summary | (R) | 4 |
| Current state | (C) | 54 |
| A + R | | 7 |
| A + C | | 11 |
| R + C | | 6 |
| A + R + C | | 4 |
| A + evaluation | | 1 |
| No comment | | 9 |
| Action instructions | | 3 |
| | | 114 |

A summary of the action taken, together with a description of the current state of the problems, was provided 11 times. Seven entries just gave a summary of the action taken. Another seven gave a summary of the action with the patients' responses. The patient's response and a description of the current state of the problem were given without mentioning the nursing action for a further six problems. Three gave instructions for future action. Only 17 forms were signed, 15 by registered nurses and two by students.

In the opinion of the district nurses 39 of 59 suggested actions could be continued in the patient's home.

| Problem | Summary/Evaluation | Suggested Action |
|---|---|---|
| Difficulty in mobilising due to swollen legs. | Walks much better but still needs supervision. | Walks with frame, encourage to use properly. |
| Newly diagnosed diabetes mellitus | Monitored blood sugar levels BM stix and urinalysis. Initially controlled by stat dose of Actrapid insulin – eventually maintained on glibenclamide 10 mg daily and diet. | 1. Advice on urine testing and diet.  2. Supervision of taking medication. |

Eight other suggested actions had been tried and had failed. For two problems the nurse said the action could not be carried out but did not explain why this was so. These were:

| Problem | Summary/Evaluation | Suggested Action |
|---------|--------------------|------------------|
| Pain | Pain from ulcer | Assessment of pain<br>*Student Nurse* |
| Inability to maintain personal hygiene | Is able to wash with minimal assistance. | Just assistance.<br>*Staff Nurse* |

When the form was first being designed the district nurses had suggested that there was a useful store of experience in nursing elderly patients in the community which ought to accompany the patient into hospital. As some of the suggested nursing actions were rejected on the basis that they had already been tried in the community and had failed, it would have been helpful and time saving if this had been known to the ward nurses.

## Problems with the Form Design

One district nurse kindly enclosed a photocopy of the summary/evaluation form with the completed questionnaire. The content had been obscured by material written on another sheet which had been placed on top of the no-carbon-required form. The ward staff had been repeatedly reminded of the care needed to avoid such a mishap. This was, however, the only reported incident.

## Opinions on the New Form

The district nurses were asked to say whether they wished to see the new form used for *all* patients transferred to their care. All but one said yes. Nineteen responses indicated it was 'better', one that it was 'generally better' and two that it was 'the same' as the old form. As the responses were anonymous it was not possible to ascertain how many district nurses had answered the question several times. The questionnaire went out with the patient and no check was kept on how many forms each nurse received.

Comments indicated that the new forms provided more information, particularly about patients' problems and treatment while in hospital:

'It is very useful to know the treatment the patient received in hospital and to know how the hospital staff view the problems that will arise on discharge home. The old forms are always very vague on suggested treatment.'

Several responses indicated that the form helped in the assessment of patients. One nurse suggested that medical problems and treatment as well as nursing ought additionally to be recorded on the form. Omissions in the information received for particular patients were also referred to, for example,

If correct information is given. This patient was not on insulin on his discharge from hospital.

Suggestions for additions to the form centred mainly on space for recording medications. The ward nurses had sometimes added a list in any unused space in the summary/evaluation section. When the form was initially designed it was thought that the transfer letter to the GP would provide this information. It later became clear that many community nurses had difficulty in obtaining access to this letter.

## THE VALUE OF LINKING WARD EVALUATION WITH DISTRICT NURSE'S ASSESSMENT

Continuity of nursing care on transfer from hospital has been the subject of repeated debate. Easy, quick solutions have been few. The early work presented at a conference on the problems of transfer home produced a flood of enquiries indicating that the proposed system appeared to have immediate validity with district nurses and their managers.

### Local Action on Findings

In discussion with the district nurses it soon became apparent that often there were problems in gaining access to the letter sent by the ward doctor to the GP. The hospital used a three-part set on no-carbon-required paper. The top sheet was shorter than the rest and did not include the paragraph about diagnosis and prognosis. This was later given in a sealed envelope to the patient to give to the GP. The other two sheets contained the full diagnosis and prognosis; one copy being posted to the GP and the other being filed in the patient's notes.

The three-part letter had the advantage that it also contained the medication prescription to be taken home by the patient. All three copies went to the pharmacy for dispensing prior to the patient's discharge. As the pharmacists refused to dispense the prescription unless the letter was complete it ensured that the junior doctor compiled the letter prior to the patient being transferred home.

The copy given to the patient for the GP was sealed in an envelope addressed to the GP at the surgery. District nurses reported that patients were understandably reluctant to allow them to open this letter. It was reported that in a small number of practices the letters were filed by the receptionist without being seen by the doctor. Access to patients' files by the district nurse was often refused so it was very difficult to find out about the patient's medication. As many of the patients in the study had disturbances of mental function the nurses did not feel they could rely on what the patient said, or on the medication containers found in the patient's home.

There was great reluctance to allow ward nurses to provide a list of the medications to be taken by the patient. The risk of transcription errors and possible litigation were the main reasons given for this reluctance. It was suggested that the simple answer was to provide a second short copy in a separate sealed envelope for the patient to hand to the district nurse. It was confirmed that a four-part set would still produce readable copies.

## CONCLUDING THOUGHTS

There is a great attraction in working with enthusiastic and knowledgeable nurses to solve long-standing difficulties and to help improve the quality of the nursing care received by patients. The researcher can gain satisfaction from knowing that an effective communication system can influence the care of many patients. In nursing there is sometimes the attitude that a nurse should be giving hands-on care not researching or managing. Having the opportunity to demonstrate that research can be equally useful adds to that satisfaction.

When analysing the data there is usually the regret that extra questions were not asked so that further information could be extracted from it. Most pieces of research finish by identifying a long list of further areas for investigation. The recent recognition that quality assurance activities are part of the proper management of the health service brings hope that much more research will be done by nurses in the future.

## References

Ashworth P (1984) People's health and their needs for nursing care, unpublished report. Department of Nursing, University of Manchester.

Barnett D (1982) *Nursing Times Series: Planning patient care – how patient care plans were designed.* 31 March.

Ward organisation – the integration of individual care plans into a work load shared by the nurses. 28 April.

The reactions of nursing staff to the introduction of care plans – adapting to problem-orientated written care plans. 26 May.

Carrying out nursing care activities – communicating and implementing nursing instructions accurately. 30 June.

A problem-orientated approach to identifying patient's problems – introducing the nursing process in the classroom. 5 July.

Corkhill B (1976) *Discharge to Community Care.* Tower Hamlets Health District, unpublished (for internal use only).

Gooch S (1988) Writing on the wall? *Nursing Times* **84**, 9, 22.

Hunt J and Marks-Maran D (1980) *Nursing Care Plans,* 1st edition. Chichester: HM and M.

Report of a Working Party of the RCN Association of Nursing Practice (1986) *Nursing Process.* London: Royal College of Nursing.

# 9
# Conclusion: Liaison in Context
## Sue Armitage

---

## THE EFFECT OF FUTURE CHANGES

Continuity of care is much more complex than its label suggests. The label itself implies something cohesive, comprehensive and easily achievable. In reality, it indicates a wide variety of service provision in variable response to the extent and quality of identified need. The entire picture, whether from hospital to home or in the reverse direction, is extremely difficult to grasp in its totality. Glimpses of the picture are seen and colour is added by a number of individuals professionally but the completed portrait remains closed from full scrutiny.

The focus on the need for continuity of care will inevitably continue to increase with shorter hospital stays. The majority of nursing demands, though, are made by elderly people and we have a burgeoning elderly population. Although the populations of most European countries are increasing relatively slowly, more than 10 per cent is accounted for by those people of 65 years or over. By the year 2000 the number of people aged 80 years or more will increase by 45 per cent (WHO, 1988). In Britain, the projected increase between 1985 and 2001 for people over the age of 75 years is 22 per cent (OPCS, 1987). The number of these over 85 years will double by the year 2001 from half a million to more than one million (Family Policy Studies Centre, 1988).

The elderly have varying needs for care. The concept of old age is changing. In the past, those over retirement age (60 years for women and 65 for men) were termed 'old age pensioners' and were considered to require additional services. That is no longer the case. In most instances only those aged 75 and over are singled out for special attention. Surveillance of the elderly does not usually extend downwards to those under 75 years. Indeed, many people over the age of 75 do not want to be regarded as being in need of services, as they think of themselves as independent. Much of the support required is that which enables an elderly person to remain or be maintained in his or her own home, such as the assurance that shopping can be obtained, and help with cleaning and laundry made available.

The changing and increasing demands for the maintenance of health care for the elderly have, of course, particular implications for nursing within the total framework of health care provision.

There have been many reports in recent years focusing on both the problems of the increasing elderly population and their needs and the place of nursing care within the provision of services. In support of the European 'Health for All' targets, it is recommended that the focus of nursing practice should be a 'multidisciplinary and multisectoral collaboration' and that it should involve individuals and their families and communities in their own care enabling them to become more responsible for their health (WHO, 1988).

Health and local authority circulars (see chapter 1) with detailed guidelines for effecting the comprehensive recommendations on discharge planning arrangements are to be commended in an area that often falls between the borders of different states. The no-man's land between hospital and community nursing and social services traversed in many instances only by the liaison sister can be a hazardous area of operation; everyone with an interest in relinquishing or taking on the burden of care but without, in many instances, the appropriate knowledge to be able to do this effectively.

The requirement that individuals should take on the responsibility for ensuring adequate arrangements for transferring patients effectively from one sphere of caring to another in a continuous manner *and taking accountability for it* will only be achieved if it is made a local requirement that is implemented. Departmental health circulars and local authorities may direct but they will not ensure changes are appropriately made and that individuals comply with recommendations made.

Policy changes in the delivery of health care have an inevitable effect on the means of delivery of local services. The opportunity for local hospitals and community units to become 'self-governing' (DoH, 1989) places a number of professional services in a previously unknown position. The predominant ideology of caring in an environment where market forces apply has distinct implications for decisions on patients' length of stay and appropriate discharge times. Where patient care is costed according to diagnosis related groups (DRG), as is the case in the US and increasingly in the UK, then a patient is most likely to be discharged after a fixed period of time deemed appropriate for treatment according to the diagnosis made. Any additional needs will probably be for nursing care, but who will provide it and in what way will be more and more of a problem.

The development of independent community nursing services following the European model (*Nursing Times*, 1989) may serve to increase patient throughput by earlier discharge from hospital for patients following certain surgical procedures, such as hip replacement. Where a standing arrangement exists then discharge procedures and follow-up care may be organised effectively. For those patients whose surgery is performed in a hospital some distance from their home, and whose home is in a district without independent community nursing facilities, the burden of caring will fall on their families and the existing community nursing services or revert to the local district general or community hospitals that have not chosen to become self-governing. The implications for ensuring adequate discharge arrangements and effective liaison are many and the consequences potentially harmful, both for the individual patient and for already hard-stretched community nursing and social services. Discharging patients who still require care into the community without adequate support is a prospect that would disturb the majority of hospital nursing, medical and paramedical staff and goes directly against the recommendations in the health and local authority circulars (HC(89)5; LAC(89)7).

## The Reality of Communication

The evidence currently available demonstrates many inadequacies in the maintenance of continuous nursing care when patients move from hospital to home. A hiatus also exists in the communication of information when patients are admitted to hospital from home where they have been receiving nursing care.

The writers who have contributed their different perspectives to this book have shown how the gap may be closed by a variety of means – either by direct collaborative discharge planning between hospital and community staff or by a designated nurse liaising between the two settings.

Groups of both community and hospital nurses are the first to acknowledge that the ideal is to have direct nurse-to-nurse communication at all times without the involvement of an intermediary. In this way they are able to give and receive the information that is most appropriate for the patient. In rural areas where community hospitals are situated and where nursing staff in both hospital and community often share the same base the ideal of direct communication and collaborative planning for patients to make a smooth transition from home to hospital and back home again can become a reality.

In urban areas and where district general hospitals serve large areas the ideal of direct communication is more difficult to achieve. Only a small number of patients discharged from acute hospital units will require community nursing services and routine channels of communication are not always established (SHHD, 1987). The lack of face-to-face contact between hospital and community nurses who have different bases and who never meet does not encourage the effort to make direct contact. Communicating confidential and sometimes sensitive nursing information about a particular patient is more likely to occur between those who have a particular name to contact and even better when a face can be put to the name.

There is also a wider gap between hospital and community nurses in larger urban areas with district general hospitals than where there are community hospitals because of the nature of nursing that takes place in each. Some smaller rural hospitals have nurse-controlled beds where the primary need is for nursing care and the secondary need for medical care provided by GPs. In contrast, in district general hospitals, where high-tech medical care is dominant, nursing care is largely in response to medical interventions and nurses have less control over their work demands. The division between hospital nurses and the nurses in the community becomes wider as they understand less about each other's role. Work experience is very different. There are fewer shared values and not surprisingly less is communicated, and often ineffectively.

The focus on nursing care in community hospitals rather than on nursing in response to the demands of high technology medicine calls for the employment of different nursing skills which can be more easily transferred between hospital and community settings. A shared nursing ideology and the movement of patients and nurses between hospital and community settings means that the division between the two is reduced and a greater understanding achieved of each other's role.

In the future, with changes in nurse education (UKCC, 1987) there will be a much greater emphasis on the preparation of nurses to work not only in hospital but equally in the community. The emphasis in nurse education will be placed on the wellness and health requirements of people as well as what they as patients require when ill. Much of the experience of students will be in the community settings where people are pursuing their everyday lives and work and where the emphasis will be one of health promotion and the maintenance of healthy lifestyles. Patients in hospital will be nursed with the recognition of them as people from within their own environment.

If this ideal were achieved, it suggests that liaison nurses will become redundant and that awareness of the community by those nurses working in hospital will be an accepted part of their role. It was thought that the National Health Service would eventually dispense with the health care demands in evidence at its inception in 1948. New demands emerged and the needs can never be met as both the consumers and the providers of health care identify still further needs and new knowledge is used to experiment with treatment and care of those who in previous generations had had no chance of survival. Even allowing for an increased awareness of what is entailed in community care it is likely that specialist liaison roles between the area of hospital and community will be necessary to provide expert advice and teaching in an increasingly complex health care system.

## Community Care, Liaison and Readmission

The work of liaison nurses and its effects are not confined to the period at or around the time of patients' discharge from hospital. There is growing evidence to demonstrate the importance of adequate aftercare and continuing community support in preventing readmission to hospital of the elderly. Contributory factors to unplanned readmission in a study of 133 elderly patients included inadequate preparation for discharge in 37 per cent of the sample (Williams and Fitton, 1988). The second most common contributory factor assessed by carers and patients was premature discharge in 58 per cent (77) of the study patients. Williams judged that readmission could have been avoided in 59 per cent (78) of patients if more effective action had been taken in five areas, one of which was 'preparation for and timing of discharge', another being 'sufficient and prompt nursing and social services support'. The remaining three areas were 'attention to the needs of the carer, timely and adequate information to the general practitioner' and 'management of medication'. Someone in the community to liaise with the hospital department, carers, formal services and GPs was recommended (Williams and Fitton, 1988).

Physical and mental stress of recently discharged elderly patients can also affect readmission rates (Brocklehurst and Shergold, 1968). Incidence and type of stress related to where patients were discharged to, the incidence rising from 5 per cent of patients discharged to live with their spouse, to 25 per cent of those going to live with a married child and to 39 per cent for those going to live with an unmarried child. Brocklehurst and Shergold emphasised the need for 'bridges between hospital and home' and comment that stress was more apparent where there was a lack of nursing and medical aftercare or where the need for 'a friendly visitor' had not been appreciated.

## The Nursing Support Interface

Townsend et al., (1988) compared the readmission rates of patients supported by a community scheme with those receiving standard aftercare. Eighteen months after discharge a significant difference was shown between the number of readmissions among those supported by care attendants in the community support scheme and those receiving standard aftercare, those in the latter group being double the number of supported patients admitted. Townsend et al., conclude by suggesting that investment in a good post-discharge care attendant service could keep patients at home and reduce unnecessary readmissions to hospital.

The services, of course, have to be available for support to be provided and care in the community maintained. Investment in appropriate services usually entails an additional commitment not only in monetary terms but in first recognising that appropriate services are needed to contribute to quality care. Benefits will accrue to individual patients but also, from the evidence cited, avoid unnecessary use of hospital services for patients who have to be readmitted because they cannot be maintained at home. The long-term and overall view of service provision is one which can be difficult to defend by service managers when immediate outlay from a hard-pressed budget is required to meet the most obvious needs at the level of crisis intervention. The idea of rationing community care goes against the ethos of nursing yet probing the detail of district nurses' caseloads reveals inadequate provision in the level of nursing care able to be given (Cottingham, 1988).

A great deal of care in the community is done by relatives, neighbours and friends. Many relatives can be taught to carry out complicated and technical procedures and many more perform what are regarded as the fundamental elements of nursing care. Controversy ranges over the nature of nursing – what it is, how it differs from caring by those who are untrained and who can do it. A large proportion of what constitutes the function of general nursing appears to be made up of activities such as bathing a patient or giving a bed pan. From an external observer's view they can be defined as simple tasks which can carry an average weighting of time for a patient of a certain level of dependency and which, it is often suggested, could be and often is carried out by someone other than a registered nurse. What cannot be observed is the simultaneous cognitive process. A registered nurse will not only be giving a patient a bedpan but will at the same time be carrying out a range of other activities, including assessing the patient's mobility, his skin condition and the level and type of interaction with him. It might, perhaps, provide the opportunity to give advice or health education, counselling or the opportunity to use complementary therapeutic techniques of caring. Last but not least the registered nurse will examine the contents of the bedpan! An apparently simple task such as enabling a patient to use a bedpan takes place within the totality of patient care and within the overall plan of care and its assessment. In this context the apparently simple provision of bathing for the elderly becomes a therapeutic activity (Nolan, 1987).

While it may often be necessary to have staff who are not registered nurses caring for patients both in hospital and in the community, it will become increasingly important for a number of reasons that any care given should be under the direction of a registered nurse. Increasing numbers of elderly people together with decreasing numbers of 18-year-olds who have in previous years provided ready numbers of nursing students are necessitating alternative approaches to adequately staffing the nursing service. Care needs to be provided in its most appropriate form whether in a combination of nursing and support services or as one or the other alone. What has to be acknowledged is the need for care to be both coordinated and adequately monitored. Primary nursing (Manthey, 1980; Pearson, 1988) enables care to be appropriately organised and delivered with the registered nurse retaining accountability for the overall delivery and efficacy of it.

Community care must of necessity be more difficult to monitor and evaluate as patients and clients are not able to be overseen together. Changing emphasis to community care demands flexibility not only in the organisation of care and its delivery but also in recognition of its increasing diversity. Knowledge of community care available and assessment of how it might best be utilised to meet the needs of patients leaving hospital and in need of continuing care is likely to become increasingly demanding, even to those nurses prepared under a Project 2000 (UKCC, 1987) programme with a much greater emphasis on community matters.

## The Consumer View

The implications of getting care right in terms of its provision, appropriateness and availability is obvious for the patient's well-being. The individual's functional capacity at home may well depend on the availability of services arranged before discharge from hospital. The effects of well-timed and appropriate provision of care and services is likely to extend to a total perception of the provision of care beyond the immediate item of care that meets a particular need. The amount of resources allocated to ensuring the provision of continuing care is likely to be relatively small within a total district or unit budget. It is impossible directly to assess in any meaningful way the amount invested against what patients receive in the way of services, their level of satisfaction and their feeling of well-being.

A support plan after discharge which is tailor-made for the individual should involve, according to Harding and Modell (1989), negotiation between the patient, informal carers and professionals rather than be solely an assessment by the general practitioner or community nurse.

## Patient Satisfaction

Patient satisfaction is difficult to measure. Structure and process features of care are more easily identified and isolated, but apart from crude mortality and morbidity figures, outcome can be difficult to evaluate. The causal link between patient wellness relates not solely to a specific intervention made but also to the complexity of total care delivered and, alongside that, a patient's general sense of well-being and feelings and perceptions about himself. An estimation of wellness is likely to be relative to a patient's previous feelings. His definition of the situation (McHugh, 1968) may well be different from a professional's assessment.

Few patients criticise outright either the medical or nursing care they receive, or even the facilities of the hospital, ward or surgery. Comments invited from patients tend to praise the efforts of nurses and indicate high levels of satisfaction (Wright, 1987). Understandably, patients are unlikely to tell nurses who ask about their opinions of care that their colleagues are thought of badly and a high degree of protection operates about 'their' nurses if patients suspect any admonition may be involved. Accurate satisfaction levels are difficult to elicit and it is crucial that the source of the enquiry is known to patients. An attempt to monitor the outcome of a programme of planned discharge of the elderly (Hunt, 1982) incorporated a follow-up of discharged patients. The anticipated low response rate (24 per cent) included only 10 per cent who expressed dissatisfaction with discharge arrangements. (The fitter patients tending to respond.)

Patients' views have not traditionally been sought and the lack of opportunity for this has in itself at times been a source of dissatisfaction to patients (Altschul, 1983). With the introduction of general management into the NHS (Griffiths, 1984) a greater emphasis was placed on consumers' views. The majority of district health authorities now have quality assurance personnel responsible for a range of quality linked developments. The way in which consumers' views should be identified, and their focus and range in terms of subject matter, will no doubt be a continuing debate.

A comprehensive survey of patients' opinions of their hospital stay has been used by a number of health authorities (Moores and Thompson, 1989). The subject matter extends from opinions of arriving at hospital, including the mode of transport, to admission and settling in the ward and views of care received. Information given and discharge arrangements are also included. Interspersed with these subjects is a large section on the 'hotel' services of the hospital and questions on hospital catering accounted for 9 per cent of the original questionnaire (Moores and Thompson, 1985).

Most consumer surveys are hospital-based. Patients in the community can only be asked to give their views on the care they receive and that generates a number of problems. Phillips (1989) states that first, and most obviously, the client in the vulnerable position of being cared for in her own home by a district nurse is unlikely to criticise the care given. Second, very often satisfaction with care and its cessation would leave a lonely old woman missing regular visits by the district nurse. Finally, a great deal of the work of community nurses is health education and promotion which may not be recognised as nursing care by the client (Phillips, 1989). Fundamental to the results of consumer opinion surveys is the understanding of the subject about which levels of satisfaction are being sought.

Patient satisfaction levels are likely to be low when there are discrepancies between what patients or clients want and what nurses think patients want. In a study on discharge planning (Johnson, 1989), 50 elderly patients rated it as 'very important' or 'extremely important' but 50 nurses who were caring for them rated it only as 'moderately', 'slightly' or 'not' important. Whatever the reasons for the discrepancy, the expressed need for knowledge and information before discharge and for patients' families to be included in planning was unlikely to be met if it was not regarded by nurses as being important to them. The need to have information early and before the point of leaving hospital was emphasised.

Patients' views of the care they received at the time of leaving hospital to return home and the preparation for it was one element in an action research study focusing on continuity of nursing care (Armitage, 1989). The first two years of the study focused on the role of liaison (Jowett and Armitage, chapter 6 this volume), the findings of which were fed into a second action research phase. In one health district three groups of hospital and community nurses and their managers, numbering about 12 in each, met together on a monthly basis. In one group there was a full-time liaison nurse and in another a part-time liaison nurse who were both health visitors. The third was without for most of the study period. In two groups, district nursing referrals were passed through the community senior nurse and one group had a designated part-time liaison district nurse. Issues of concern to both hospital and community staff in ensuring continuity of care were identified and examined within the action research cycle. Within each group interventions were planned and changes then implemented and evaluated (Lewin, 1946; Susman and Evered, 1978).

Nurses' perceptions of the efficacy of changes made were measured over a period of time by a questionnaire. Patients were interviewed in an attempt to establish an outcome measure for the process of assessing, arranging and organising aftercare. All too often, professionals feel they know what is best for their patients without asking them, although many nurses cannot easily articulate what patients want other then in general terms. Patients (N = 76) were interviewed at home 7–10 days after discharge and asked about what they considered to be important to them at the time of leaving hospital and returning home. In general, the patients were extremely accepting of the services offered and their levels of satisfaction high; the corollary being that their levels of expectation were low. As this study was carried out in an area a deprivation in the South Wales valleys it is perhaps not surprising that the level of satisfaction should be different from the elderly patients from a central London group practice (Harding and Modell, 1989). The inhabitants of a deprived social area have often only ever known a scarcity of services and adjust their expectations accordingly. On the other hand, many people enjoy within the 'valleys community' of such an area a degree of family support which is lacking in an inner city area. While recognising that the elderly generally express more satisfaction than those who are younger, Harding and Modell (1989) found that a third of the 115 patients they interviewed were dissatisfied with the notice of discharge they were given. In the action research study (Armitage and Williams, 1990) in many instances elderly patients were only too glad to go home and either were not concerned about minimal notice of discharge or would decide to go home immediately following a consultant's ward round. It was much more likely to be a relative who expressed the view that a little longer notice would have given more time to prepare for the person coming home.

An individual patient's perception of satisfaction and well-being is entirely subjective. The professional assessment of a patient at home with dyspnoea and an oxygen mask might well be different from that of the patient. In answer to a question on how he was feeling and being given the choice of a seven-point range of responses from 'very well' through to 'very ill' one patient in this situation insisted he was 'very well'. In probing this further he said he was in his own home with his wife. His grandchildren could call and see him; he was very well.

Quality care by definition must take account not only of the consumer's varying levels of expectation but also meet professionals' agreed standards. Yet, to be realistic, quality care cannot be provided as the 'ideal' care possible in the best of all possible worlds. There are inevitably the constraints of the resources available and quality care is often the optimum care possible within those available resources. However, more emphasis may be placed on providing efficient nursing care than on providing quality of care. 'Care can be delivered efficiently, but not necessarily at optimum quality' (Abdellah, 1984). Professionally assessed patient care may be of a high standard. If patient and client needs are taken into account patient care is likely to be even better and what is more, the patient is likely to be more satisfied as well.

## The Hospital and Community Powerbase

'Liaison' is used as a single label but it is not a single entity. The term 'liaison nurse' can be used to describe a full-time district nurse or health visitor, who may assess patients individually or enable and facilitate patients' assessments by hospital nurses. 'Liaison nurse' can also be used to describe the clerical 'half a day a week' activity of calling into hospital wards to collect names and addresses of patients referred for community care and passing them on to colleagues for visiting. Melia and Macmillan (1983) describe the different levels of importance attached by district nurses to liaison depending on whether or not they had ever done it themselves. Liaison in reality includes multiple facets of communication and contact between hospital and community and at times, many individuals. Under the specific label of 'liaison' its complexity disappears.

In the future, community nursing may hold a different place in the balance of power from the present one. The majority of nurses currently registered started their nursing careers in hospital and even for district nurses, hospital nursing was to them, initially, the normative version of nursing. 'Hospital dominance means that hospital nurses and doctors do not think in community terms' (Melia and Macmillan, 1983: 63).

An action research study focusing on continuity of nursing care and involving hospital and community nurses in regular face to face contact (Armitage and Williams, 1990) showed that a 'linkage hierarchy' currently operates (see Figure 9.1).

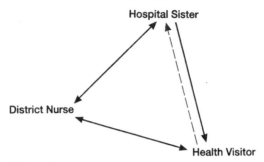

**Fig. 9.1   Linkage hierarchy.**

The hospital sister at its head sees herself as readily available and at the end of a telephone in a health care system dominated by a technologically-oriented hospital environment. Communications between hospital and community nursing services are usually concerned specifically with the continuation of general nursing care and unilateral in direction. Far fewer communications go in the opposite direction from district nurses to ward sisters. Occasional enquiries by district nurses for information on a particular patient cannot always be handled by the ward sister and with shorter working weeks hospital nursing staff may not have background information on a patient who has been admitted and discharged during their off-duty days. This is likely to happen increasingly with faster throughput of patients and shorter hospital stays.

Yet at the head of the hierarchy the dominant position of the hospital is maintained. Telephone communications to one hospital through another's switchboard compounds such hospital dominance and difficulty in communication. It is certainly the case that district nurses with a community caseload are likely to be easily accessible only at certain times of the day when the telephones at their base are also likely to be busy. Few district nurses have car telephones, long-range bleeps or even answering machines at the surgeries where they are based (Edwards, 1987).

District nurses and health visitors communicate with each other in varying degrees, largely depending on whether or not they share the same base. Their degree of understanding of one another's role and function is increased by their both being community nurses although their is often an element of rivalry in the appropriateness of one or the other assessment necessary.

Health visitors and hospital sisters rarely, in general, communicate with each other. Many hospital-based nurses do not understand the role of health visitors, especially in relation to the elderly (Melia and Macmillan, 1983: Armitage, 1989). Confusion arises between the function of health visitors and social workers and when it would be appropriate to refer patients to the health visitor on discharge from hospital. Rarely is there any communication from a health visitor to the hospital staff. The dominance of hospital over community is compounded.

## IN CONCLUSION

Ensuring continuity of nursing care is no easy matter. The chapters in this book reflect 'reality' to those doing the job of day-to-day patient continuing care. The problems they experience and how they have overcome those problems are perspectives from where they stand, on one side or the other, that so often divides care in hospital from care at home. In chapter 5, a view of the community hospital is given where barriers between hospital and community staff are few and where care can often be contained within a revolving door policy. In many instances this is not possible. An effective liaison service needs to be built on the sound provision of a service that does not detract from an individual practitioner's skills, abilities and experience but where it can add to it (chapters 2 and 4). Chapters 3, 7 and 8 have described ways through the hazardous terrain of the no man's land of post-discharge care, showing how things can be made to happen successfully and problems surmounted.

The importance of flexibility with statutory and voluntary services provision is likely to increase as health care and education changes take effect. Coordination of those services is vital. In the future we may have a nurse able to work effectively in hospital and community alike. To do that, boundaries between the two will have to become much more flexible.

Continuity of care is an area of concern that will not go away. There is a great deal of evidence to suggest that it is not yet right. Whether it is with the development of nurse-to-nurse communication or through an intermediary liaison nurse for each individual unit decisions need to be taken on the method most appropriate to thats' particular situation. Whichever system is chosen it will be important to monitor and evaluate it in the constantly changing situation in which health care is delivered.

# References

Abdellah F G (1984) Overview of the quality of nursing in the US, paper presented at the Quality Assurance Conference, UMIST, Manchester.

Altschul A T (1983) The consumer's voice: nursing implications. *Journal of Advanced Nursing* **8**, 3, 175–183.

Armitage S K (1989) Liaison nurse: the key to continuity of care. In *Good Practices in Community Nursing*, Monograph No. 2. University of Manchester, Department of Nursing.

Armitage S K and Williams L (1990) Liaison and continuity of nursing care. Unpublished research report.

Brocklehurst J C and Shergold M (1968) What happens when geriatric patients leave hospital? *The Lancet* **2**, 1133–5.

Cottingham M (1988) Rationing community care. *Nursing Times* **84**, 11, 16–17.

Department of Health (1989) *Working for Patients*. London: HMSO.

Edwards N (1987) Nursing in the Community – *a Team Approach for Wales*. Review of community nursing in Wales (Chairman Noreen Edwards). Cardiff: Welsh Office.

Family Policy Studies Centre (1988) *An Ageing Population*. Fact sheet 2. London: FPSC.

Griffiths R (1984) *NHS Management Inquiry Report*. London: HMSO.

Harding J and Modell M (1989) Elderly people's experiences of discharge from hospital. *Journal of the Royal College of General Practitioners* **39**, 17–20.

HC(89)5 (1989) *Discharge of Patients from Hospital*. London: Department of Health.

Hunt M (1982) An action research approach to promoting planned discharge of the elderly from acute wards to the community. In *Proceedings of the RCN Research Society XIII Annual Conference 1982*. Durham: University of Durham.

Johnson J (1989) Where's discharge planning on your list? *Geriatric Nursing* **10**, 3, 148–9.

LAC(89)7 (1989) *Discharge of Patients from Hospital*. London: Department of Health.

Lewin K (1946) Action research and minority problems. *Journal of Social Issues* **2**, 34–6.

Manthey M (1980) *The Practice of Primary Nursing*. Boston: Basil Blackwell.

McHugh P (1968) *Defining the Situation. The organization of meaning and social interaction*. New York: Bobbs-Merrill.

Melia K M and Macmillan M S (1983) *Nurses and the Elderly in Hospital and the Community: A study of communication*. Report prepared for the Scottish Home and Health Department, Nursing Research Unit, University of Edinburgh.

Moores B and Thompson A (1985) From the patient's mouth. *Health and Social Service Journal*, 22 August, 1040–2.

Nolan M R (1987) The future role of day hospitals for the elderly: the case for a nursing initiative. *Journal of Advanced Nursing* **12**, 683–90.

*Nursing Times* (1989) Community pilot scheme slammed. *Nursing Times* **85**, 9, 7.

Office of Population Censuses and Surveys (1987) *1985–2025. Population Projections* London: OPCS.

Pearson A (ed.) (1988) *Primary Nursing: Nursing in the Burford and Oxford Nursing Developments Units*. London: Croom Helm.

Phillips K (1989) The myth of consumerism in the NHS. *Primary Health Care*, April, 14.

Scottish Home and Health Department (1987) *Nursing Issues, Priorities and Action in Scotland*.

Report of a nursing colloquium held 2-3 April.

Susman G and Evered R (1978) An assessment of the scientific merits of action research. *Administrative Science Quarterly* **23**, 582-603.

Townsend et al. (1988) Reduction in hospital readmission stay of elderly patients by a community-based hospital discharge scheme: a randomised controlled trial. *British Medical Journal* **297**, 6647, 544-7.

UKCC (1987) *Project 2000: A new preparation for practice*. London: UKCC.

Williams E I and Fitton F (1988) Factors affecting early unplanned readmission of elderly patients to hospital. *British Medical Journal* **297**, 24 September, 784-7.

World Health Organisation (1988) *Summary Report*. European Conference on Nursing, Vienna, 21-24 June.

Wright S (1987) Consuming interests. *Senior Nurse* **6**, 2, 24-6.

# Index